The Politics of Dietary Change

MICHAEL MILLS
City of London Polytechnic

Dartmouth

Aldershot · Brookfield USA · Hong Kong · Singapore · Sydney

Published by
Dartmouth Publishing Company Ltd
Gower House
Croft Road
Aldershot
Hants GU113HR
England

Dartmouth Publishing Company Ltd
Distributed in the United States by
Ashgate Publishing Company
Old Post Road
Brookfield
Vermont 05036
USA

A CIP catalogue record for this book is available from the British Library and the US Library of Congress.

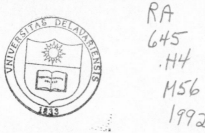

RA
645
.H4
M56
1992

ISBN 1 85521 226 9

Printed and bound in Great Britain by
Billing and Sons Ltd, Worcester

Contents

Acknowledgements

This book is based on a doctoral thesis written at the University of Essex between 1985 and 1990.

Many people have made contributions to this book in one way or another. In particular I would like to thank my parents and brother for keeping us mobile, looking after the children and for the food parcels; my mother-in-law for paying the car tax, loaning the money for my computer, taking the children and giving us much-needed holidays; my father-in-law for his generosity, the trips to Shetland, the whisky, and the chocolates; and Grandma for the cheques which seemed almost endless, and which eased things considerably.

Academically, the list grows even longer. The interviewees who gave me their time and attention were promised anonymity and so cannot be mentioned by name. Nevertheless, I would like to formally acknowledge their contribution to this work, and thank them for their insights and comments which were often invaluable.

I must also thank the staff and students in the Department of Government at the University of Essex for their interest in, and contribution to, my work. I would particularly like to thank my supervisor, Hugh Ward, who has shown great faith and trust in me and Dave Marsh, Rod Rhodes and Tony Barker who have all taken a great interest in my academic prospects and gone to a great deal of trouble to foster and further them.

Three other people deserve a special mention. Mel Read has been exceptionally kind in both his help with word processing, and the many discussions we have had on health, prevention and policy communities. Mike Saward has given me the support of a good and valued friend and this has often been what I have needed most; and Rob Stones has given me the benefit of his many thoughtful and perceptive insights.

Undoubtedly though, it is my wife (Bunny) and children (Rebecca, Emily and Hannah) who deserve the greatest thanks.

My wife's unfailing strength and loyalty have made it possible for me to continue and to hope for success. Without her strength and her love, the whole thing would have been unthinkable. To my children I can only offer my apologies and my love.

Mike Mills, May 1991.

1 Introduction

In recent years there has been a great deal of consumer and media concern about food and health. Some of the issues that have been raised, such as Listeria, Salmonella and Botulism, are questions of food safety and contamination. Others, such as food additives and food irradiation, focus primarily upon what is deliberately put into food, or the processes it goes through before it reaches the consumer. In all these areas, there are legitimate concerns over the foods available and their contribution (or otherwise) to health.

Having said this, the publicity surrounding these issues is, in many ways, disproportionate to their ability to adversely affect the health of consumers. This is not to say that certain food additives are not carciogenic, or cannot cause hyperactivity. Rather, while these issues may be symptomatic of general problems within the British food chain they are not in themselves the greatest danger to the public health.

It is known (for example: WHO;1982. BMA;1986.), that there are structural problems with the diets of western countries generally, which predispose Westerners to particular diseases. Diets which are high in salt, sugar and fats, and low in fibre, are correlated with high incidences of tooth decay, obesity, cancer of the bowel and colon and high blood pressure. However, by far the largest diet-related health problem in western countries is heart disease which, in terms of diet at least, is primarily associated with fat intake.

In Britain, heart disease is responsible for approximately 180,000 deaths per year and is the single largest cause of death (DHSS;1981, Smith and Jacobson;1988,p29). This in itself may be sufficient to justify a study of the political responses to the problem, particularly since heart disease has been a major cause of death in Britain since the 1930's. Thus, heart disease is not only a major health problem in Britain it is also the major health consequence of western diets more generally. Furthermore, there is evidence to suggest that while the incidence of heart disease has shown dramatic falls in other countries (notably, the USA, Australia and New Zealand) the fall in Britain came much later and is much less dramatic (CPG;1986. Interdisciplinary;1984). This also requires an explanation.

But a study of heart disease is also interesting and justifiable because it is the only diet-related health area which has something resembling a policy attached to it. By this I mean that the problem has been officially recognised, the present government has accepted some responsibility for its solution and there have been some policy initiatives. In 1984, the British government accepted a report from the DHSS's Committee on the Medical Aspects of Food Policy (COMA) which contained a number of recommendations to government on how to reduce the incidence of heart disease through changing the diets of the population (DHSS;1984). By looking at the responses of the government to those recommendations, the broader forces which shape the food supply and the diet and health debate can also be considered. In short, a justification for this study would look to the number of deaths attributable to heart disease, the apparent difficulties that Britain has been experiencing in reducing the prevalence of the disease, the possible economic consequences that such a reduction would entail and the challenge that health professionals have presented to the British government.[1]

---

[1] I should mention at this point that the terms "state" and "government" are not used interchangeably. When "state" is used it refers either to consistent features of the apparatus' of government through time regardless of which government is in power, eg. the state's commitment to agricultural support, or, to a collection of governmental institutions at a particular point in time, eg. the challenge that health professionals have presented the British state. The term "government" is used when referring to those things which are specific to a particular government, eg. the government's response to the COMA report.

Methodology

There are certain conceptual problems with focussing attention on only one part of a much broader debate and, in many ways, this study necessarily falls between two larger issues. Heart disease is a multi-factoral disease, that is, it can have a number of different causes, of which diet is one. Equally, the relationship between food and health is based upon a wide range of political and economic variables of which fat in the diet is one. It is necessary to make clear, therefore, that this study is not intended to explain all policies on either heart disease or food and health, only the intersection of the two. Having said this, diet and heart disease does represent perhaps the most important of the issues which touch upon "nutrition" in the population and as such provides a relatively self-contained study within the broader debate.[2] Given that a study of the whole field is impracticable, this case is representative of the others and draws, where possible, on illustrative examples from them.

The reasons for addressing the problem of diet and heart disease at all have come from circumstantial evidence which suggested that there were political and economic reasons why the British government has (1) been reluctant to embrace the new dietary evidence, and (2) has been primarily responsible for the persistence of high levels of heart disease.

Originally, this evidence came from Walker and Cannon's book *The Food Scandal*, in which they argued that a report by a government-sponsored committee on diet and health was "suppressed" because of its commercial implications (Walker and Cannon;1985). Given that the arguments surrounding food are invariably concerned with its health consequences this suggests that there is some degree of political conflict between contending interests within this policy area. Thus, the focus of this study is to establish what has been the basis of the government's response to this issue and how it might be possible to account for known policy outcomes.

To test this, on one level at least, is a relatively simple exercise. Given that the government accepted a report by health professionals on this subject the obvious strategy would be to compare the recommendations made by the professionals to the policies that emanated from the government. If they bore little resemblance to each other, then it could be argued that professionals had not been influential and that politico-economic

---

[2] Important in terms of morbidity and mortality.

considerations could be important.

In many ways, though, this approach would over-simplify both the political circumstances surrounding the acceptance of the COMA report and, indeed, the methodology that the study requires. The COMA report was an honest, but not particularly radical document with a narrow policy focus. Methodologically this has advantages and disadvantages. The major disadvantage is that it is not necessarily representative of the broad cross-section of professional reports on diet and health. The primary advantage, of course, is that it was accepted by the government and can be seen as a point of reference against which government polices can be measured.

Now, the government's response to the 1984 COMA report is clearly crucial to any test of what it's calculations were, but I would argue that it is not sufficient. There needs to be an attempt to establish what the opinions of health professionals are on the question of diet and heart disease and this needs more than the recommendations of one report. In other words, one example is insufficient, a representative sample of the available reports needs to be taken; I have done this in Chapter Three.

The other over-simplification which could come from a straightforward comparison between "recommendation" and "response" is that it implies that if the government acts in a way which is consistent with the recommendations of health professionals it does this only because it is responding to those recommendations. Clearly, this assertion needs to be qualified because it ignores, for example; the ability of health professionals, or other groups, to place issues on the political agenda; other societal forces which can produce a political response for other unrelated, reasons; and it also ignores the motives and intentions behind the government's responses. Despite these shortcomings I would argue that this methodology is the only reasonable one. The major objections which can be raised to it revolve around the difficulty in *measuring* the effects of political actions, or discriminating between one source and another. Neither of these are problems if it is possible to establish why the government is acting in a particular way and what its calculations are. However, it does mean that it is necessary to distinguish between simply creating the political climate in which the government believes it must do something and establishing how much difference that climate has actually made to the resolution of the problem under consideration.

However, the greater part of this study is taken up with trying to provide an explanation of why the policies that emerged after the 1984 report (*Diet and Cardiovascular Disease*) take the form they do.

Empirically, there is no single reason why this should be the case.

4

Walker and Cannon's argument that economic interests within MAFF have effectively blocked new policies on diet and health certainly provides part of this explanation but by no means all of it. This type of argument cannot, for example, explain why the Department of Health (DoH) should acquiesce to such pressure from another Ministry, nor why MAFF appears to act as the agent of a sectional interest at the expense of the public health. Simply considering a government's response to one report at one point in time will not, therefore, provide the evidence necessary to understand the role of professionals or to explain the other forces involved in policy making and implementation.

This requires an historical consideration of what policies, principles and assumptions have under-pinned the relationship between the two departments and the relevant policies within each. In this way, it is possible to establish what the state's historical role has been with regard to the food supply, what the persistent features and characteristics of the policy area have been and whether, ultimately, these are part of an explanation of policy outcomes. I will argue that they are crucial to such an explanation.

Theoretically, the same problem applies. The key distinction remains the two sides of the policy area; food and health. A theoretical characterisation of the forces involved has to achieve three things. Firstly, it must account for the power of professionals, because it is largely their power which is being tested. Secondly, it must explain why decision making and representation within MAFF appear to exclude professional opinion and privilege food interests. Thirdly, it should provide a framework for discussing the above as a single political structure, so that meaningful comparisons can be made between food and health.

Research Problems

The research problems have stemmed almost entirely from the topicality and sensitivity of the diet and health debate. It has not always been possible to gain access to the people or the documentation that would have been most useful. This was particularly true of government officials and representatives of industry. When this access has been forthcoming it quickly became clear in interviews that interviewees were invariably reluctant to talk freely about "health" issues. Most interviewees were assured that our conversations were confidential and that any information I used from them would be unattributable. Hence, I have not identified them beyond giving their profession.

Most difficult of all, however, has been the tendency amongst government officials and industry representatives to be reserved about their contacts with each other. All industry representatives, without exception, were sensitive about discussing their links with MAFF, or indeed, other sectors of the industry. The impression was given that they wished to play down their relationship with MAFF, and few would commit themselves to saying how often they dealt with MAFF, on what issues, and with whom they dealt.

With an area such as this there is little that has been published and one of the few ways to establish patterns of relationships and policy preferences is in interview. Given the reticence of interviewees, it has been difficult to establish the processes which constitute the formulation of policy and the specific considerations that interested parties (particularly MAFF) attached to the various options available. This is a theoretical as well as an empirical problem. The current trend in network theory (which I shall be using in this study) has been toward disaggregation (see, for example, Wilks and Wright;1987) and establishing the detail of the political processes which produce policies. I am not unsympathetic toward this trend, and wherever possible, this type of approach has been adopted. However, in the absence of the information necessary to take that approach, the alternative is to consider policy outcomes rather than policy processes. Obviously, there are disadvantages in doing this because it relies upon inferring from known decisions and eventual outcomes what the intentions of the policy were at the outset. Needless to say, there is no necessary reason why there should be strong correlation between intention and outcome.

Having said this, I would argue that it does not present insurmountable problems. With the exception of some details, which can be explained in terms of the idiosyncrasies of particular governments, policy outcomes are historically highly predictable. Certain features of state action throughout this century are very consistent and suggest that its intentions have been, and are being, realised. It is not only historical continuity which suggests that policy outcomes are deliberate because the policies of the 1980's show the same trend. For example, there are at least three cases of government-sponsored publications relating to diet being delayed, edited or suppressed by the government since 1983[3]. In cases such as this it is impossible to

---

[3] The NACNE Report (HEC;1983), the JACNE leaflet (HEC;1985) and the COMA report on the diets of schoolchildren (Wenlock et al;1986).

6

disaggregate because, by definition, they are politically sensitive. Nevertheless, it is still possible to draw insights and inferences from these examples particularly when they are consistent with other historical and institutional data.

The Chapters

This section looks at the sequence of, and arguments in, the following chapters. Its purpose is simply to outline the structure and organisation of the book and, in some instances, to justify the approach adopted.

In the following chapter I introduce the theoretical concepts I will be using to explain the policy area. This chapter is not intended to provide explanations itself, this is the job of Chapter Eight , its purpose is simply to explore the concepts I wish to use, and to present some of the problems I believe exist with them.

These concepts come very broadly from two schools; one is network theory, and the other is the literature on structure, power and agency. There are a number of reasons for choosing these above others. Firstly, network theory appears, at first sight at least, to be able to characterise the areas of food and health very accurately. The control that MAFF has exerted over food policy could be, and has been, described as a "policy community" which can exclude other (consumer) interests from decision making. Secondly, network theory can also characterise and explain the power of professionals to the extent that they can be seen as a "professionalised network" (Rhodes;1986). Within this single theoretical approach, then, two contrasting patterns of political relationships can be accommodated.

Chapter Two does identify some problems with network theory which I attempt to resolve. In essence, this case study looks at the effects of change within a policy area, and this is something that the literature on policy communities does not address satisfactorily. Consequently, when I discuss and define policy communities, I emphasise how and why they may adapt to the changing political environment in which they find themselves.

The basic contention of these contrasting characterisations of professionals and the interests within MAFF is that the distribution of their power resources is such as to advantage those within MAFF. Given this, it is argued that network theory has to be supplemented by some account of the nature of the resources available to agents and the structures through which those resources are used. Rhodes' idea of "resource dependency"

7

goes some way toward this, however, as Stones has argued, Rhodes does not go far enough (Stones;1988b). Resource dependency cannot distinguish satisfactorily between structural and non-structural resources, and is not clear enough on what distinguishes "resources" in decision making from "constraints" on it. Because of this a more precise account of what structural power actually is and how it exists through time is extremely useful in helping to understand how networks and communities emerge, and how they change.

Chapter Three places the issue of diet and heart disease in its professional context and is divided into two parts. The first part looks at the evidence which links diet to heart disease and argues (1) that there is a broad professional agreement on the evidence, and (2) that heart disease is a problem in Britain. Obviously, both of these points need to be established if a study of the influence of health professionals on this subject is going to be meaningful. Clearly some degree of agreement is required before a political response might be expected to the recommendations of professionals and equally, the existence of a problem is a prerequisite for the adoption of a solution to it.

The second part of the chapter looks at how the problem of dietary change and heart disease has been tackled in two other countries, the USA and Norway. These countries differ in the approach they have taken to the disease. In the USA, it is the medical profession which has taken the lead, while in Norway, it seems that the state has been more active in promoting dietary changes. In many ways this reflects the differences in their political systems and it is the relationship between system and response which is one that will be used explanatorily in Chapter Eight (Theoretical Explanations). Finally, again in Chapter Three, I try to summarise the recommendations contained in several eminent medical reports on what the principles of a policy on diet and heart disease might be. I have stuck to principles, rather than specific policy suggestions, firstly because the reports are not all at Britain and secondly because, numerically, they are far more manageable. There are four policy principles which appear to be central; (1) The policy must be preventive in nature; (2) it must be a national policy with local initiatives;(3) it must be consistent and (4) it must address the whole population, not simply those at risk.

Schematically, it is essential to know what professionals are suggesting, and which approaches have been adopted in other countries before any consideration of the historical background to Britain's policies. The purpose of the following chapters is to characterise British policy in the areas of food and health (generally termed nutrition). Much of the significance of this characterisation would be lost without knowing (1) how it "fits" with current nutritional orthodoxy or (2) how it might be implemented.

Chapters Four, Five and Six are historical. By looking at nutrition policy since targeted (and characterising briefly the pre-war period) it is possible to see a number of underlying principles and assumptions which conflict with current dietary advice. For example, it becomes clear that while the state will encourage supply during peace time it is extremely reluctant to interfere directly in demand; even though, logically, the former could be said to presuppose the latter. The only exception to this is when there is a threat to food availability (ie, in times of crisis) such as the World Wars, the depression, or the recession of the early 1970's. Clearly this is an important structural feature of the policy area which conflicts with current dietary guidelines which infer a stronger role for the state in directing consumption. Similarly, the role of the market in food supply, the power resources of professionals and the curative nature of the health service all have historical roots which have been institutionalised in the British political system and all have some bearing on policy outcomes.

By the end of Chapter Six, therefore, we should have the major elements of policy, the division of responsibility that exists between MAFF and the DoH and the constraints that agents and policies must take into account. In this way, both the opinions of professionals that were outlined in Chapter Three and the subsequent account of the policies pursued in the 1980's will be more readily understood.

Chapter Seven is a straightforward account of what the British government has done in response to the 1984 COMA report on *Diet and Cardiovascular Disease* which deals with the main policy initiatives and evaluates what the calculations of the government have been. It is argued that while professionals have placed the issue of diet and heart disease on the political agenda they have had far less influence over the policies that emerge. Indeed, the response of the government is consistent with the historical principles of policy which favour personal responsibility, rather than state action, and the protection of a competitive market in food. Chapter Eight returns to the theoretical concepts outlined in Chapter Two to provide an explanation for this. The core problem has been the shifting scientific paradigm surrounding nutrition. The previous paradigm, had been the scientific basis for much post-WWII food policy. When this shift occurred, changes in those policies were inevitable. Having said this, the change has not been in accordance with professional opinion, and it is this resistance to change which then needs to be explained.

This is done by looking at the ability of the policy community within MAFF to control policy procedures and the inability of professionals to apply their resources outside of the confines of the NHS. Equally, the division of responsibility between MAFF and the DoH, the role of the market in food supply and the entrenched positions of commercial interests within MAFF are all structural features of the policy area which contribute to the final policy outcomes.

*   *   *   *   *

In essence, this book is about change and the resistance to change. It deals with a changing scientific orthodoxy, the changing political pressures that arise from this and the reluctance of political institutions to respond to change. But it is also about those features of our political system which persist, sometimes for very long periods, despite the changes in the rest of society. The tensions that result from these two contending positions reveal not only what is central to the policy areas under consideration, but much of what is axiomatic to the British political system more generally.

2 Theoretical Perspectives

From the *Introduction* I hope it is clear that any attempt to explain the dietary change policy area in theoretical terms will need to accommodate a range of empirical variables. The views of health professionals are clearly going to be one of these as will the structure of, and relationships within, the health service. But there are other factors which are equally important. The relationship between health professionals and the Ministry of Agriculture, Fisheries and Food (MAFF) is also important to the extent that MAFF is responsible for many of the measures which may reduce heart disease. Equally, the relationships, values and policy orientations within MAFF and between MAFF and other groups will, in turn, explain their response to professional attempts to advise on coronary heart disease (CHD). In each of these cases it is necessary to explain and account for the variables individually and in relation to one another.

This needs theoretical concepts which can explain at both the macro level and at the meso-level. At the macro-level I will use structure and power as over-arching concepts to "join together" the policy areas of food and health and the relationship between professionals and food interests. At the meso-level I will look at professionals, professionalised networks and policy communities.

11

I will argue that structure and power can be seen as a means of conceptualising relationships across policy areas and that the notion of structural power and relative resource advantages within and between structures is a useful and accurate characterisation of this case study. While professionals are indeed powerful their power is not necessarily politically sufficient for their own purposes, and it varies depending on what type of professional we are looking at. The pattern of relationships between professionals is described as a professionalised network, and this is contrasted with the concept of policy communities, in which power is more concentrated and membership less numerous; policy communities and policy networks characterise the nature of decision making within MAFF very well. Finally, these concepts are drawn together under the umbrella of structure and power to show how they can coherently accommodate the primary relationships, values and policies of this case study. The application of these concepts to explain particular policy outcomes is not the subject of this chapter but is dealt with in Chapter 8 (Theoretical Explanations).

Structure and Power

The literature on "structure" is extremely diverse and if it shares any common feature at all it is simply that authors disagree with one another. Indeed, Lukes (Lukes;1978, p9) has gone so far as to say that he believes structure to be an essentially contested concept in the same way as freedom and equality have never been consensually defined. The label essentially contested presents the danger both of avoiding useful concepts and of becoming a self-fufilling prophecy. Each of these dangers can be avoided by clearly stating the meaning of the concept as perceived by the user; this is largely the objective of this section.

It is probably easiest to begin by defining what is meant by the term structure and follow this with a detailed explanation of it.

A structure is defined and distinguished by a set of mutually adjusting relationships, the standardised expression of these relationships and varying potential for action.

I will take this definition bit by bit. In alluding to a set of mutually adjusting relationships I am largely following Giddens'[1] (Giddens; 1978,p69) contention that relationships are what he calls "recursive"; that

---

[1] And Lindblom of course.

is, each time a person interacts with something or someone, the structure is in some sense reproduced, although not in the same form. Relationships are at the core of structure; this is not to say that agents are simply bearers of structure, but rather, that a part of what is structural exists abstractly between agents in their interaction, their perceptions of their own position and the positions of others. I also agree with Giddens (1978,p56) that these relationships change through time, that agents adjust their actions because of the circumstances in which they find themselves. If, for example, I pursue a course of action which, in my terms, does not succeed, then I would, in all likelihood try something different next time. If I succeed the first time under one set of circumstances, but those circumstances change, then it would be sensible for me to adjust my actions accordingly if I ever wanted to repeat the previous outcome or one which was equally favourable to me. These relationships are "mutually adjusting" because if I am sensible enough to change my actions, then it must be expected that in response to this, others will do the same, either with regard to me, or someone /something else which is affected by my actions. The most obvious example of this would occur when two people (sides) were negotiating and had to adjust their respective responses continually. Of course, the essence of recursion is that it happens everywhere, not just in these formal situations.

Where I disagree with Giddens, and with Marxist and Neo-Marxists concepts of structure, is that I believe that structure can and does have a material form. This is the essence of the second part of the definition which refers to the "standardised expression of the relationships". Going back to Giddens for a moment, his characterisation of the fluidity of structure is revealing and intuitively plausible because recursion is something we all do all the time. What appears to be lacking in Giddens' account is why some aspects of society, in the broadest sense of the word, change very little through time. Even things which might be viewed as undesirable, such as inequalities in health care provision, the relationship between disease and social class or poverty do not seem to lend support to the idea that structures are typically fluid to any great extent. This is particularly important for Giddens because he, unlike structural Marxists (Benton;1984. Carnoy;1985), is reluctant to give great significance to ideology as a feature either of structure or the social system (1978, p71-72). He therefore has less opportunity to explain those things which are persistent through time and which adversely affect large sections of the population.

By arguing for standardised expressions of relationships I am saying no more than that the everyday operation of "mutually adjusting relationships" can and do have material consequences which become part of the structure

13

itself. At any given moment in time "things" are being created which express the relationships which exist at that time. These expressions are standardised in that they will remain constant in their form unless deliberately changed, unlike the relationships themselves. They can also be taken as meaning standardised in the sense that they express a standard form of the structure as it existed at the time of its creation. The National Health Service is a good example of this. The structure of the NHS is the product of many past adjustments between agents, ranging from the early choices between central government funding and basing the system within the auspices of local authorities, through to the present proposals for NHS reform. The consequences of this have been that the physical arrangements of the service, as well as its principles, were established and have remained until they were altered. In other words, a universal health system, free at the point of delivery, is an expression of a past political event (mutual adjustment) and it is also a structure in the same way that doctors and nurses are a structural feature of the NHS.

Before I deal with the last part of the definition, I must take a brief look at the concept of power as it can be used in this framework.

I want to draw primarily on the work of Lukes and Ward here and argue that power is the capability to achieve a desired result, and that the exercise of power is the exercising of that capability. To exercise power implies four things:

1. That there is a deliberate and conscious act (intentionality) (Lukes;1978,p6) - although this does not mean that you necessarily intend the outcome of your actions.
2. That there is a choice available to the exerciser, that is, that the exerciser is to some extent free to act and his or her actions are not structurally determined. In this way it is possible to attribute responsibility for actions (Lukes;1978,p6 and 1984,p21).
3. That there is a relationship between exerciser[s] and subject[s].
4. That there will be an effect that would not otherwise have come about.

As Lukes point out, this applies to non-actions as well in that I can exercise my power by doing nothing and still produce an outcome. Power in the sense I am using it should be seen as the utilisation of structural and/or non-structural resources; that is, resources are the "vehicles" (Giddens;1978, p69) of power and power can only be exercised through them.

The final part of the definition of structure refers to the varying potential for action. By this I mean that power, as the capability (potential) to achieve the result that is desired, is, by definition, unevenly distributed throughout structures. In other words, there will always be those people or interests that are more powerful than others. I recognise that there may well be examples of societies in which this was not the case, in which it was never accepted as the norm, and that there may well be, in the future, structures which are egalitarian and which have a more or less even distribution of power within them. What I am arguing is that all the structures of which I am aware and which I am interested in are asymmetric in their relations, hierarchical in their organisation and have a "varying potential for action".

This varying potential for action refers to a power-capability that can best be seen as the ability to draw on resources. These resources are then employed by the agent in a way which s/he believes will further the ends they have in mind. Indeed, Giddens (1978,p63) argues that it is through resources and rules that structure should be defined. In a sense this is what I have done by speaking of varying potential for action. But there is an important difference between Giddens' use of the term and mine.

I want to argue that structures provide resources which may be drawn upon by agents, as would be the case when the decision was taken by the DoH not to publish, for example, a report by the National Advisory Committee on Nutrition Education (NACNE). Only those agents who had the resources to publish the report could be the ones that refused to do so. That, to me, is the exercise of structural power, ie. the utilisation of structural resources upon a circumstance for a desired end. Giddens argues that all power is structural, that because action and structure presuppose one another, and because all resources are structural, then as a consequence, all power must be structural. I would follow Ward (1987,p598) however and argue that there are such things as non-structural resources and hence non-structural power. Ward gives the example of barristers (Ward;1987,p599) who vary in their rates of success not only because of their varying structural resources but because some barristers are simply better than others; this has nothing to do with structure at all. Another example is that of the Chief Medical Officer (CMO) of the DoH, Sir Donald Acheson. It has been argued (Street;1988) that the government's response to AIDS has, in large part, been the result of the personal (non-structural) qualities and values of the CMO in addition to the obvious resources that any CMO would have. In short, his structural location and the circumstances within which he worked could not provide any adequate account of his behaviour.

In fairness to Giddens he can account for this difference between individuals through the idea that each person interacts with structure differently because of their different life-experiences, but that ultimately, because structure is the resources and rules that govern agency and most of our consciousness, then these resources and hence potentials must, for Giddens, be structural. The problem here, of course, is establishing causality; which particular life experience, which particular structure is responsible for the action we are interested in?

An obvious consequence of the uneven distribution of resources within structures is that the ability to achieve preferred outcomes within that structure, and perhaps others as well, is concentrated rather than dispersed. This can mean two different things. Its most obvious meaning is that power (resources) are concentrated in a particular place in the structure, so that, for example, the higher up a hierarchy we go, the more resources we would expect to find. However, it could also have another meaning which focuses on particular agents who are not "concentrated" in a spatial sense, but their power is nevertheless concentrated within them as a class of agents. Doctors are the most obvious example of this. The resources that they apply in their relationships with their patients are reasonably consistent between doctors and so it is reasonable to argue that power is concentrated within doctors, even though they are not, as a group, all roughly in the same place.

The fact that some people or interests are more powerful than others does help (structurally) to explain the rather obvious problem of things persisting through time which are generally unpopular. This still leaves the problem of accounting for change. On one level this is easily done because I have argued that by definition structures are mutually adjusting, and hence one would expect them to be changing all the time. On another level the response must be more complex. Radical change in the structure appears to contradict my contentions so far to the extent that dominant structural forces might be expected to retain their position, and the structure itself, through the utilisation of their resources. This may indeed be the case, although this may not necessarily be their explicit motivation, merely an unintended consequence of their actions. So, if there is uneven distribution of power in structures, why is it that sometimes these structures change radically to the disadvantage of those who have most power?

Part of the explanation comes from the fact that these structures should not be seen in isolation from each other. Given that there are many co-existing structures at any one time which may operate relatively autonomously it can be argued that what is structural for one person is not necessarily for another. Equally, what is structural for one person at a point in time, may not be at another time. For example, the Minister of Health

16

can, in principle, change the whole nature of the structures within which the health service operates from outside even if it is impossible for any internal coalition within the NHS to affect radical change.[2] So, an internal coalition is constrained in a way which a Minister is not.

This is one explanation whereby greater resources are applied to a given structure from outside. Another explanation would look to the workings of the structure itself, and may focus on the interaction of mutual adjustment and standardised expressions. If mutual adjustment amounts to the source of constant change within a structure, then standardised expressions are the opposite; they express beliefs, relationships, ideas from the past or the present. They are not dynamic in themselves but can be used as a source of dynamism inasmuch as they may be utilised by agents and can be changed, although generally not easily. They prevent the rampant fluidity of structure by providing resources; they are in a sense anchors of the structure in a particular configuration. Yet there are a number of possible ways in which these anchors (standardised expressions), and the uneven distribution of resources may be insufficient to maintain the structure in a given configuration. There may, for example, be the unintended consequences of action which inadvertently deprives the dominant forces of resources or provides other sections of the structure with resources. It is certainly the case, for example, that the introduction of the Poll Tax had the unintended consequence of raising individual payments above a politically acceptable level in some parts of the country. Consequently, the government lost resources in terms of their authority and legitimacy as well as the obvious costs in terms of public expenditure. Another way would be that mutual adjustment was in effect drawing the structure towards certain orientations or commitments which were incompatible with the resources or standardised expressions of the dominant forces. For example, the Common Agricultural Policy is a standardised, structural variable which is increasingly seen as being anachronistic because the agricultural needs of Britain, and the prevailing political climate have changed gradually through time so that there is now a tension between the CAP, the government and the means of implementing agricultural policies. A still further example is simply that new resources are accumulated which destroys the previous distribution of power potentialities. For example, environmental groups such as Greenpeace and Friends of the Earth have developed their own resource bases and pools of expertise on nuclear safety and water purity which, to them, is a new resource which changes the nature of their

---

[2] Thanks to Hugh.

relationship with the government. There may also be changes in how agents perceive their own interests which would also alter the utility of present structures and resources, or, actions may become constrained by structures through time which prompts the desire to change those structures.[3] In short, through time a person, or groups, interests may change and their ability to get their own way may also change.

This is not an exhaustive list of those things which may cause structural changes, but it does demonstrate I think that it is possible to identify both reasons why structures may exhibit certain continuities through time, but also why they may change by degrees, or radically.

I will conclude this section by reiterating some of its major points. The definition of structure used here interprets the concept as having both an abstract and a material form which may be utilised by agents. It allows for the constraining and the facilitating of action by the structure and by the utilisation of the structure. It sees the resources within the structure as being unevenly distributed, and, while it does not necessarily imply predominance or asymmetry within the structure, this is likely. The relationship of this to dietary change will be made clearer later in the chapter.

Policy Communities

The reason for bothering with policy communities at all is that it provides a label for a certain type of decision structure which appears to be prevalent within the policy areas of food and health. Policy communities exist both in MAFF and the DoH and, because of their integrated nature, exert a powerful influence over policies. Rhodes (1988) argues that policy communities are groups that are highly integrated, exclusive, stable, have resource dependencies within them and generally have resource distributions which favour the state over other participants in the community (ie. they are uneven). It is not difficult to see that, on Rhodes' account at least, this fits with the ideas on structure, agency and power I gave in the previous section. I argued, for example, that within a structure, in this case a policy community, power would be unevenly distributed; I also argued that power would have to be exercised through resources and this also fits with Rhodes' model of power-dependency, that is, that political relationships are based upon the exchange of resources in a more or less dependent way. Equally, the stability of a policy community could also be anticipated given the fact that it is a structure which has a relatively

---

[3] Thanks to Hugh Ward for these last two examples.

18

concentrated level of resources (compared with those outside of it) which in turn should be capable of manipulating those resources to its own advantage through time.

The concept of a policy community can therefore be used as a label to describe the particular configuration of a structure. By this I mean that it can help us to distinguish between those who make decisions and those who do not, those who have dominant resources and those who do not; and, in conjunction with the broader concept of "networks", it can help distinguish between one type of decision making structure and another.

Structure, power and agency are also explanatorily important because they provide the link between action (agency) and the collective interests of the community itself. They can account for the calculations of the members of the policy community and can explain the interaction of the community with other societal forces. This type of account is conspicuously absent from the existing literature. I will return to this later.

For the purposes of this study the labels that are used to describe the political relationships within the field of dietary change are extremely important because many of the relationships are very complex. To provide a full theoretical account of the motives, actions and policy outcomes it is necessary to incorporate into a framework at least six politically distinct interests, groups of interests or political actors; farmers, food manufacturers, health professionals, technocrats, and the political and administrative staff of the MAFF and the DoH. Within these groups there are also sub-groups, for instance, different sub-sectors of the food industry. The question arises, therefore, of the extent to which the concept of policy communities will be helpful in characterising any, or all, of these political relationships? Firstly, though, we have to establish what they are. Rhodes has argued that policy communities are a:

> ..response to the imperatives of rationalisation and the
> changing socio-economic circumstances of government.
> (Rhodes;1985,p16)

They are a means of decision making that has developed because the state has assumed greater responsibility for the functioning of society, particularly in the post war period. The areas of food, agriculture and health are all classic examples of this. Richardson and Jordan (1978) argue that this has brought with it "sub-national government" whereby decision making shifts off the minister's desk and into policy communities or policy "sub-systems" (1978,p115). Wright (1987,p20) wishes to "reserve" the term for the lower level of the policy sub-system and it has been widely used as a concept applied to the study of centre-local relations (Rhodes;1986. Rhodes;1987.Sharpe;1985) and government-industry relations (Wilks and Wright;1987. Grant,Paterson and Whitson;1988). Similarly, Rhodes (1986,p26) has argued that policy communities should be confined to what Lindblom has called "ordinary" rather than "grand" issues .

I would argue, however, that it is the particular relations within policy communities that are of explanatory importance not their spatial location. Of course, location may be important in terms of the members' (agents) abilities to draw on structural resources, but this should not be taken as meaning that policy communities exist only where the centre is weak. The existence of policy communities should not be taken as an excuse to argue for a pluralist model of decision making in Britain (Jordan;1981). Defence procurement (Gray and Jenkins;1985), Health Authorities and Agricultural price support negotiations are all examples of policy communities which exist at various levels of the political system. If policy communities do exist in central government, then it is not necessarily the case that they are only concerned with "ordinary" issues. It seems likely that this type of configuration of relationships would suit even "grand" issues. Thus, I would argue that decision making structures that might reasonably be called policy communities can be found at any level of state activity.

The definition of a policy community that will be used here has five central characteristics. These are; (1) they have a particular field of authority and responsibility; (2) there will be predominant actors within the community, that is, power will be unevenly distributed throughout the membership; (3) the membership of policy communities are relatively stable through time; (4) this membership has a consensus on policy values and hence (5) it will exclude those who do not or will not adhere to such values.

Again, it is possible to see the compatibility between this definition and the definition of structures in general that I gave in the previous section. The relationships within the policy community revolve primarily around (1) the power resources afforded by the structural position of agents both as members of the policy community (eg. authority, legitimacy) and as members of related structures (eg. the resources that the NFU might bring to a policy community - expertise, representational authority, financial resources) and (2), the perceived interests of the membership. Similarly, it is possible to see that the consensus on policy values represents an adherence to particular ideological commitments. The compatibility should come as no surprise because a policy community is part of a structure itself, thus, what applies to one must apply to the other.

There are some marked differences and similarities between the definition I have given here, and those that can be found elsewhere. As I said earlier, Rhodes' definition is close to the one I have used here, as is Laffin's (1986). Wilks and Wright, on the other hand, use the concept differently. They argue (1987,p296-305) that these communities are simply the pool of interests and potential interests who have "a common policy focus" (1987,p299). There are two points which follow from this. The first is that a policy community, for Wilks and Wright, can, presumably, have a very large membership if it includes all those interests who may, potentially, have the same policy focus. This is in contrast both to the ideas I have expressed here, and those to be found in Rhodes which see policy communities as a having a small membership. The second, and more important point, is that Wilks and Wright appear to argue that policy communities are not decision making structures in their own right, but rather, provide the clientele for policy networks which are then the location for decision making.

Now, the useful thing about Wilks and Wright's ideas on communities and networks is that they see them as separate entities which can co-exist. What is far less useful, however, is the idea that these communities can have large memberships and that they do not make decisions. As Rhodes and Marsh have pointed out:

> ...there seems little advantage in turning the concept of
> "policy community" on its head. Virtually every other
> author treats policy communities as highly integrated
> ...personal networks (Rhodes and Marsh;1990,p18).

It should be noted that there is no logical reason why we cannot accept that communities and networks are both personal networks of some description and yet also accept that they exist simultaneously. I would agree that a policy community should be seen as being integrated and exclusive, and also that it will have a network of relationships within it; this is inevitable in any structure. However, I see no reason why this policy community cannot establish networks which service it and which are far less integrated. It seems quite reasonable, particularly given my arguments on structure and power in the previous section, to view a policy community as only one part of a larger structure, but a part which has certain distinguishing (definitional) characteristics. Because of the nature of these characteristics the policy community would control much of the structure of which it was a part. In this way there may be many networks and communities within policy sub-sectors and it would then be possible to plot them more precisely. This is precisely how I see food and farming interests interacting with MAFF. There is clearly a dominant policy community which involves MAFF and the NFU but this exists in conjunction with a series of sub-central policy communities and networks which have a greater input from food manufacturers. Empirically, the need to have communities and networks existing simultaneously is, therefore, very important for this study. I will return to this point when I consider networks in more detail.

Some aspects of this definition do not appear to contradict much of the existing literature. Having a consensus on policy values (or an agreement to differ on certain aspects of policy), uneven resources, a certain field of responsibility and a stable membership are all fairly uncontentious in terms of the existing literature. The feature which is far more contentious, however, is that the *exclusion* of alternative values (or ideologies) is definitional. Exclusion can take two forms which I have called *ideological exclusion* and *overt exclusion*. Ideological exclusion occurs when a policy community (or, indeed, a network) tries to prevent those outside of the community from formulating alternative policy values. For example, in Chapter Six, I will tell the story of the NACNE report which was an expert report on diet which was suppressed by the DoH. This is ideological exclusion because it prevented the formulation of ideas by the general public which the publication of the report would have afforded. Overt exclusion comes when these values already exist but are simply not given an input into policy by the community. This can range from simply ignoring those (unacceptable) opinions, through to incorporating them only partially and hence depoliticising an issue without actually conceding anything. This has happened with the 1984 COMA report on *Diet and Cardiovascular Disease*. The extent to which this will be the case, and the extent to which this is politically justified, will be a matter for empirical investigation, and will, of course, vary between policy areas. There is no given level of exclusion just as there is no given level of integration in a policy community. The need to exclude these opinions represents a desire on the part of the policy community to continue to make policy in a particular way and towards particular ends, after all, that is the primary reason for there being policy communities in the first place. Exclusion is definitional, therefore, to the extent that a policy community will exclude alternative value orientations if they have been politically articulated and activated; this does not preclude the possibility that these alternative orientations do not exist politically.

As it stands, the literature on policy communities and policy networks has managed to provide labels for particular structural configurations, and to give these structures certain characteristics but there are other things which need to be labelled and accounted for. Firstly we want to know about the internal workings of policy communities. Secondly, we need to characterise how policy communities deal with the many interests which are affected by its actions in the broader political environment.

The characterisation is straightforward. Policy communities and networks have both an internal and an external environment similar in nature to the three environments identified by Laffin (1986). Internally, there will be a cognitive paradigm based upon the values of the policy community, the rules that govern participation and the knowledge that each member has of the other members, for example, in terms of the resources at their disposal. These features of the policy community contrive to create stability both in the relationships that exist and in the direction of policy that emanates from it. Taking the policy community in isolation, therefore, it is not difficult to see how stability and consistency of outcome might be expected because there is a lot of agreement and understanding between the membership.

It is far more difficult to characterise the environment which is external to the policy community as having this degree of stability. While communities exist to control policy in a consistent way, the external environment is subject to many forces and many ideologies. This environment can be comprised of interest groups, individuals, other policy communities and networks, in fact, any interest which is affected by the policy community. In an attempt to be a little more specific, however, I would argue that for our purposes we should concentrate on those interests which have been *activated* and which are participating in the political process.

It is not unreasonable to suggest that the potential for dynamism is far greater in the external environment than it is within the policy community itself. There are fewer features of this environment which anchor it toward certain policy orientations, in fact you would expect a great number of competing interests with strong opinions on what the policy community should be doing. In terms of food and agriculture policy that is an accurate description of the situation in the 1980's but for most of the post-war period there was a high degree of consensus between those inside and those outside MAFF on what policy should look like.

23

Unlike the past, the relationship between the policy community and its external environment now has to be manipulated in such a way as to create only minimal levels of tension between it and those interests it effects. The process of ideological exclusion is one way of doing this, of course, but less malign methods would include making concessions in sensitive areas of policy, undertaking research on certain aspects of policy, setting up committees of enquiry etc.

Now, these relations can be seen in terms of the mutual adjustment of relationships between agents within a structure. In the previous section I argued that all relationships were recursive, that is, we are all adjusting our relationships with each other all the time. In this sense, no structure can be entirely immobile; a policy community may be stable and consistent but it is always adjusting its relationships within itself and with other external forces.

A policy community can be seen as a collection of agents interacting with each other to provide a consistent and deliberate effect elsewhere in the structure they inhabit. The membership of the community apply their resources (exercise power) in order to do this, and in so doing, enter into a relationship (recurse) with others. The resources they apply can be either structural or non-structural. The product of this action, from the policy communities point of view, should be the maintenance or generation of their preferred policies and the manipulation of the external environment so that this is possible, ie. minimising unnecessary tension.

This, then, amounts to the *process* which is absent elsewhere; it is an account of interaction based upon ideas of structure, agency and resources which are distributed in a particular way. *Change*, or to be more precise, the need for change, can then be seen as an inevitable consequence of these processes. The extent of this change will depend upon how well the policy community controls the policy area. Policy communities are always changing but will try to avoid being forced into changes they don't want to make. For example, the reason why there is a debate about dietary change is that in the past policies have been pursued which have solved some problems (under consumption) but generated new ones (heart disease, for example). There has been a relationship between policy and consumption but it is only relatively recently that the effects of the policy have been discovered. Consequently, a number of structural changes have occurred. One is that there has been a change in the perceived interests of certain groups in the external environment and hence a change in their relationship with the communities and networks surrounding food and farming. Another effect has been a change in the distribution of resources. The knowledge of

24

the health effects of past policies is a new resource to those who oppose current policies, and hence the distribution of power has now changed. In the previous section I gave other examples such as the application of greater resources from outside the policy community by, for example, another policy community. Changes in policies, therefore, have to be explained in terms of (1) the distribution of resources within or between structures and (2) the perceived interests of those who inhabit the structures. This account allows us to plot the relationship between the actions of the policy community through time and the effects that those actions have on all structurally related interests; it provides an explanatory tool with which to approach the existence of, and changes in, policy communities.

The importance of this for our case study lies in the fact that diet and health is a policy area which is in a state of flux. Policy makers, particularly within MAFF, have been under a great deal of pressure from consumer groups, the media and health professionals to change their policies in line with new scientific evidence. Hence, while the agents who make policy have not changed, the circumstances under which it is made certainly has. Similarly, while the decisions being made now are consistent with those of the past in terms of general orientation and values, the way one would characterise those decisions has also changed; they are no longer based upon a consensus. In these respects, the model I have presented can provide explanations.

There still remains the problem of giving a fuller account of what a policy network actually is, and of how to incorporate professionals into our analysis. This is the subject of the following section.

Professionals

Health professionals are important for two reasons. Firstly because they are the primary bearers of the new knowledge of nutrition and hence have resources which are politically significant. Secondly they are generally seen as a powerful group which, again, makes them politically important. These reasons suggest that the role of health professionals in policy making and implementation could be crucial in terms of public policy and its effects on public health. Consequently, this section looks in some detail at the sources of professional power, the cleavages which may exist within the health profession and ultimately at the best way to characterise professionals theoretically.

Until relatively recently the literature on professionals has come almost entirely from sociology and has centred around two main approaches. One is "trait theory" in which a profession is distinguished from a non-profession through its particular characteristics or traits. These usually include such things as a common body of knowledge or training; working practices which are licensed by law; professional control over recruitment; a shared professional ideology and authority over the occupational field.

The other approach has seen professions as functional in their attributes so that the "traits are only those which have functional relevance for society as a whole." (Johnson;1972, p23). More recently however, the question of professional autonomy has been seen as definitionally crucial (Johnson;1972). Autonomy, not only comes from the traits of a particular profession, but from the field in which the profession operates and the wider socio-economic and political variables which affect that field (Illsley;1980.p60).

Johnson (1972,p45), for instance, argues that it is the professional's ability to manipulate the "tension" or "uncertainty" between themselves and their clients which will determine how autonomous they are. Friedson (1970,p84) also sees this autonomy as residing in the profession being able to determine the form, if not the content, of their work.

There are a great many problems with this concept because of the variety of specialisations, locations and clientele that need to be accommodated into any one definition. Laffin, speaking of professionalism, forwards the idea that it is a:

> ...peculiar type of occupational control rather than an expression of the inherent nature of a particular occupation (Laffin;1986,p21).

Here again, we return to "autonomy". Even so, this control will be peculiar to the occupation itself for reasons which are self-evident; not all occupations are the same. Friedson appears to agree:

> In the case of professions, autonomy apparently refers most of all to control over the content and terms of work. That is, the professional is self-directing in his work (Friedson;1970,p134).

This autonomy is also achieved, for Friedson, by the "formally created position of a profession". This is done through institutional (political) means which gives "authority" to the behaviour and opinions of professionals. In turn, this extends the range of things that need to be considered as integral to a profession to include the formal or official aspects of professions and professionalisation.

The conclusion must be, therefore, that a profession will have certain characteristics, that it is primarily defined in terms of the autonomy or control that it has over its work and that this autonomy is owed, in part at least, to some form of licensing by the state.

There are certain problems with this approach which are particularly evident when considering the role of professions with regard to public policy. One of these problems is that once a profession has been established, I would argue that it's autonomy is maintained through a continuing process of service provision, ideological generation and political activity. In other words professions must protect their professionalism by doing their job and reminding the state of how useful they are. Secondly, it seems that the possession of knowledge by professionals, particularly technical knowledge, has been underplayed. The ideologically binding effect of this knowledge and the barriers that this creates between professions and non-professions (particularly politicians) are both politically important. Thirdly, and perhaps most importantly as things stand, the power of a profession is measured in terms of their relationship with their clients, rather than with reference to wider political variables. These variables may include such things as legislation (and the ability to influence it), as well as budgetary decisions, procedural rules and the like. I will deal with these in more detail a little later on.

A distinction needs to be made between the autonomy that a profession has over its clients and the power that it has to maintain that autonomy. Laffin makes a similar distinction through his three autonomies over work, self-regulation and policy (Laffin:1986,p23). The reasons for such a distinction are the same here in that professions not only provide a service to their clients, but also have a political role. For example, the removal of the household conveyancing monopoly from solicitors; the deregulation of opthalmic prescribing or simple changes in public expenditure can all affect professions and can amount to a test of their power or influence which has very little to do with their relationship with their client. In other words, professionals have to continually create the conditions under which they can retain occupational control.

How might they do this? What might be the limitations of their influence over public policy decisions which may be of interest to them? Dunleavy (1981,p10, also see Dunleavy 1982) is interesting on this point. He contends that a primary resource of a profession is ideology. He argues that professions may generate ideologies in the peripheral agencies of the state which are subsequently ratified by the centre. He further says that at the "substantive level" of policy making there may exist "ideological corporatism" which is an integration of organisations worldviews through the professions.

Clearly there is much truth in Dunleavy's assertion concerning the profession's ability to create ideologies which exist not only in professional networks but also in policy making arenas. The medical profession is a prime example which has been said to have created a "hegemonic situation" (Saunders;1984) within the health service in Britain. But the assertion cannot go unqualified. Dunleavy says that "eccentric" behaviour is likely to be counter-productive in terms of professional influence and this suggests that the "rules of the game" are not determined by the profession alone. Equally, at the "substantive" level (which is presumably in central government rather than its agencies) professional ideology is only one of the necessary requirements for effective political action, indeed, it may be only one of many ideologies. It cannot be assumed therefore, that the existence of a unified professional outlook will always allow for professional influence over policy.

Similarly, this suggests a number of other points that need to be made. The first is that there are not only the opportunities for the permeation of professional ideology into centres of decision making, but also for the building of relationships, the routinisation of consultation and the continuing input into policies. Secondly, professional access will be issue-related, and will be specific to the needs of the decision makers and/or the profession. Thirdly, and as a consequence of the above, professional input into policies will, unsurprisingly, be confined to their specialisation. Equally, there may be intervening variables which dilute the potency of this base. For example, an issue may straddle a number of policy areas, it may be politically contentious, the policies may be economically significant or perhaps need solutions which are radically different from previous policies. In any of these scenarios, a professions influence may be less than might otherwise be expected. In short, there are any number of reasons why professionals may not be powerful at all, and these reasons may be missed if we focus entirely on the relationship between professionals and their clients.

The Elite/Professional/Technocrat Cleavage

From the above, it seems clear that there are important political features of health professionals; the fact that they bear knowledge is obviously one of these, as is the fact that they have a similar ideological outlook. These features, which would tend to homogenise professional action, belie the fact that within professions there are many different sub-groups which may compete with each other. For example, from this case study it is possible to demonstrate a number of different groups, each of which could quite reasonably be subsumed under the heading "health professional"; nutritionists, dieticians, GPs, consultants, professors, nurses etc . Some of the distinctions which could be made are politically important, and some are not.

For the purposes of operationalising the definition I have only distinguished between elite professionals and health professionals, that is, the rest of the professionals. I have done this primarily because, within the latter group, I have found empirically that there are no noticeable differences in their attitudes towards the evidence on diet and heart disease nor is there any perceivable conflict between these groups in areas which relate to this case study. The only possible qualification to this could come from the trade-off between, for example, increased resources in cardiology, and the resources available for heart disease prevention. This, in turn, would reflect differences in interests within the group I have called health professionals. While these intra-professional conflicts may exist, it is difficult to establish any clear demarcation lines which would help in identifying a distinct sector of the profession and which would, as a consequence, add anything of explanatory value to the case study. This is not to say, of course, that in other case studies, useful distinctions could not be made.

It seems to me that the most useful distinction that can be made comes from distinguishing between professionals, elite professionals and technocrats. These distinctions are useful because each group has played a different role with regard to diet and heart disease. I will begin with technocrats and move on to make comparisons between them and professionals and professional elites.

Bell (1976) defines a technocrat as "one who exercises authority by virtue of his technical competence". Laffin (1986,p23) argues that within the state there are both public service professionals and those whose role is "techno-bureaucratic" in nature. The apparent intention of both authors is to identify those who have both technical competence and authority. This suggests that the following may help to distinguish a technocrat from a professional:

1. A technocrat combines a managerial and technical role and has work goals organisationally defined. A professional has fewer managerial responsibilities and greater control over work definition.
2. The application of a technocrats' knowledge may be mediated by

alternative ideologies or open to lay interpretation. That is, the knowledge may be manipulated in some way before it is applied to the problem. Professionals would apply knowledge in a less mediated fashion.

3. Technocrats are not only subject to professional ideology, but also to bureaucratic or other extra-professional forces (which may be ideological or economic in nature). This may affect the formulation of opinions and the advice which follows.

4. As a consequence of this technocrats may have a "dual loyalty" (Massey;1985,p9) or be inclined to put "emphasis on the organisations own interests" rather than those of the public or the client, in a way which may not be the case with professionals (Dunleavy [a];1981,p198).

5. Technocrats are unlikely to be as dynamic as professionals in the generation of new knowledge and ideologies. This is because their own knowledge is defined by the needs of their employers and thus may be "localised" and out-dated (Johnson;1972. Dunleavy [a]; 1981,p197).

It will never be possible to draw a perfect line between professionals and technocrats. Whole branches of a profession may be considered technocratic in some way; top corporation tax barristers, for example. On the other hand, there is obviously no given level of ideological interference or knowledge mediation by bureaucratic organisations. Equally, it should not be assumed that professional opinions reflect some objective truth or that being employed by an organisation necessarily means that a persons integrity is compromised.

Politically, the distinction is very important for our purposes. In this study there are three primary sources of information and knowledge available to governments and their decision makers. One is the professional elites which includes a variety of specialisations (cardiologists, nutritionists, dieticians) and it might be expected that their authority and knowledge would provide resources which enable them to influence policies. A second source is the food industry which employs and/or retains experts whose knowledge is relevant to the needs of the industry itself. The difference between these "technocrats" and the professional elites is simply that their clients are different; the technocrats are answerable to their Director or Chief Executive. Whether this makes a difference to the advice that is given or to the knowledge that is generated is a question that will be tackled later. A third source, also technocratic, are the civil servants within government who are employed because of their expertise. Those who are significant in this policy area reside in the Scientific Divisions of MAFF and in the DoH. They provide opinions and interpretations on information

30

for the departments they serve which is then utilised not only according to "scientific" criteria, but also according to political and economic criteria as well.

Let us return to the distinction between the bulk of professionals and the elites of those professions. Clearly they will share a great deal in common; ideology, training, certification etc, but there are also differences that are politically important. To begin with, elites within a profession may be established in peak organisations to further the interests of the profession. In this respect, it is easy to distinguish between representatives of the British Medical Association, for example, and a GP. But the elites are not only those in the peak organisations, they are also those eminent in research. Hence the British Medical Journal could say that "doctors sensed a battle between the experts" on the evidence relating diet and coronary heart disease (BMJ;1984,p509). The distinction was implicitly made between those who administer knowledge and those who generate it. It is generators who are "experts" as well as professionals and who are to be found on government advisory committees. Few if any of these people are practising professionals in the usual sense of the expression. They are unlikely to have the usual clientele of patients, but rather, spend much of their time researching. By a professional elite, therefore, I simply mean those who represent either the "sharp" and "expert" end of the profession or those who represent both the knowledge and the profession. Etzioni-Halevy defines an elite as:

> ...minorities of people who are especially influential in shaping society's various institutional structures or spheres of activity. (Etzioni-Halevy; 1985,p15).

On this definition, which I think is broadly correct, it is reasonable to include "representatives" and what Etzioini-Halevy calls "intellectuals" in the expression elites because of their influence over the institutions and professions themselves. The distinction between technocrats and elite professionals remains largely the same as that between professionals and technocrats in that one would expect elites to retain a much greater degree of autonomy over their work than technocrats.

Now, the political utility of knowledge is that it is a scarce resource and the bearers of it are, in essence, claiming authority for their opinions because they know something that other people do not. Medical and scientific knowledge is particularly prone to this sort of interpretation. The implications are that a group (health professionals for example) will claim authority over a policy area because they know best. Increasingly, however, this expectation becomes unsustainable as the possible sources of knowledge and advice increase, not least within government itself. In consequence, the power of professional elites to achieve their policy objectives may diminish because governments and decision makers have multiple sources of advice each of which claims to be correct. Another consequence of this is that it removes the uncertainty between the professional and their clients' (in this case government). Anyone who ignores a doctors' advice does so at their own risk, that is, they are not in a position to judge what the consequences will be and therefore are largely obliged to comply. Having a second or third opinion available which offers a different option presents the client with choices and the confidence to defy the doctor because the consequences are more fully understood. This scenario is one in which the influence of the doctor is diminished because of the existence of alternative opinions, and that influence would be further reduced if those alternatives were more in line with what the client actually wanted to do. In other words, the advantage that is usually enjoyed by professionals is the clients uncertainty about what will happen if they do not comply with professional advice. Again we return to a scenario in which we have to qualify the power of health professionals (in our case elites) this time because they are in competition with technocrats.

Communities, Networks and Professionals

We have already looked at policy communities in some detail, and have seen that they are integrated, exclusive structures which have responsibility for decisions within a particular area of policy. Before we move on to consider how this helps to characterise health professionals, elites, and technocrats I must spend some time considering what a network might be and how it can be distinguished from a policy community.

Rhodes argues that the term "network" provides a useful metaphor for policy making and implementation structures. Following Benson (1982) he defines a network as a:

> ..complex of organisations connected to each other by resource dependencies and distinguished from other clusters or complexes by breaks in the structure of resource dependencies. (Benson, in, Rhodes;1986,p22)

These networks will vary along five "key dimensions": constellation of interests; membership; vertical interdependence; horizontal inter-dependence; and the distribution of resources (Rhodes;1986,p22-3). It is Rhodes contention that these networks take various forms, for example, policy communities, territorial communities, producer networks and professionalised networks. For Rhodes, therefore, a policy community is a type of network. In general, then, a network would be seen as a more open structure (entry qualifications excepted) with power dispersed rather than concentrated. Issue networks, which surround particular issues within a policy area, are even less integrated. Thus, Rhodes sees these networks "ranging along a continuum from highly integrated policy communities to loosely integrated issue networks" (Rhodes and Marsh;1990,p6).

On this basis it appears that the main feature which distinguishes, for example, a policy community and a policy network, is the degree of integration. I take "integration" to mean, for example, the extent to which the agenda of a policy area is controlled by a given number of actors, the breadth of value orientations that can be accommodated, the entry qualifications for participation, the extent to which the "rules of the game" are malleable etc. This, of course, differs from Wilks and Wright's conception to the extent that they believe the membership of a network will be drawn primarily from that network's policy community.

I agree with Rhodes that the level of integration must be the primary variable which helps us to distinguish between policy communities and other types of network and that these networks do give greater opportunities for broader participation. Having said this, I think that one has to be careful about the degree of latitude in policy that this infers. It must also be remembered that any network is a structure, and as such, must share a great deal in common with policy communities, as Rhodes recognises. It is the similarities, as much as the differences, which are of explanatory importance. There will still be recursion and mutual adjustment, an uneven distribution of resources, varying potential for action and standardised expressions of the relationships within the network. The basis of the interaction between the agents within networks should, therefore, be seen as differing from policy communities along those criteria which define structure itself. Thus, one would expect those within a network to deal (mutually adjust) with a greater number of other interests (in terms of absolute numbers or range of interests); that resources would be more evenly distributed, and so power would be more evenly spread. Of course, this has to be seen in context. Resources will still be unevenly distributed, the state is still likely to retain a strong negative capability and there is unlikely to be rampant fluidity in policy orientation.

I do not want to use the term network in the sense that Wilks and Wright do, and ascribe to it any necessary decision making function. A network is, first and foremost an observable pattern of people concerned with policy. Of course there are different types of network, professionalised and producer for example, but this implies that policy communities and networks can co-exist. It is perfectly possible, under this characterisation, to have a policy community which controls most major aspects of policy which is serviced by a professionalised network or which is formed by part of such a network. Despite the degree of political control exercised by a policy community this could still allow the development of issue and policy networks around the less important aspects of policy.

Other models provide a range of possible ways to characterise professionals, elites and technocrats. A professionalised network, according to Rhodes is:

> characterised by the pre-eminence of one class of participant in policy making - the profession....In short, professionalised networks express the interests of a particular profession and manifest a substantial degree of vertical independence whilst insulating themselves from other networks. (Wistow and Rhodes;1987, p 8)

Wilks and Wright, on the other hand, argue that:

> ..the National Health Service is not one policy network, but a policy community with several policy networks for, for example, the family doctor service, and for mental health, hospital, and maternity services. Whether or not these networks are professionalized will depend on the extent to which the medical profession, or parts of it, has a dominant role in each (Wilks and Wright;1987,p302).

When Haywood and Hunter looked at decision making within the DoH (rather than the NHS) they argued that policy was made in "iron triangles" (Haywood and Hunter;1982).

There is a grain of truth in all these perspectives. I think that to ignore the fact that within the health service health professionals are predominant would be an oversight and would ignore the consistencies that appear to exist in professional behaviour. There is no reason why, at this aggregate level, this cannot be called a professionalised network and should not be given the characteristics suggested by Rhodes.

Having said this, it is clear that policy communities (according to my definition) do exist within health authorities at regional and local level and, given that the membership of these communities is partly drawn from the professionalised network, it is necessary to see professionalised networks as operating at the sub-central level partly through these policy communities.

Similarly, it would seem more appropriate to characterise the relationships which exist around the Units within the DoH as policy communities, rather than iron triangles, if for no other reason than to achieve some terminological consistency. This does not seem inconsistent with the arguments forwarded by Haywood and Hunter.

In this way, therefore, health professionals within the health service could be described as being part of that professionalised network, but may belong to other networks and to policy communities as well depending, for example, on whether they were members of the boards of health authorities. It would then be possible to disaggregate the category of professions further, if the policy area suggested this was necessary.

If this framework is used I think that it can help to explain the continuing need to reproduce the conditions under which professionalisation can flourish, because it extends the focus of professional interest out of the work place and into policy communities. Thus, it is possible to argue that the extent to which professionals will be able to preserve their autonomy will depend upon their success in controlling those institutions which affect their workplace. Similarly, their success in securing their policy preferences (whether these enhance autonomy or not) will depend upon their success in establishing themselves within the communities and networks which actually make policies.

Elite professionals can be seen in the same way. They may constitute an elite network within a particular specialisation of the profession or around core institutions such as the DoH or the BMA, for example. In other words, they may service part, or all, of the profession. Similarly, there is no reason why they cannot constitute part of the membership of a policy community or an issue network. The primary differences between an elite network and others are the nature of the membership and the political roles they are likely to have. Thus, the membership of an elite network is far more likely than other parts of the profession to be coopted into decision making processes at central level. This also tends to give elite networks an enhanced authority because of their degree of expertise and because, in most cases, they are seen as representative of their profession.

Having said this, it is necessary to qualify it by returning to a theme I have already mentioned. An elite network is elite within its own domain, that is, only in comparison to the discipline from which it is drawn. There is, therefore, no necessary policy *effect* that can be implied from the existence of elite input into public policies. Furthermore, the existence of an elite does not necessarily imply that an elite network exists, it is quite possible that elites will act individually and idiosyncratically, without reference to any broader network. Whether a network exists, will, of course, be a matter for empirical investigation.

Technocrats present different problems however. There is evidence to suggest from this case study that agents who display technocratic attributes can constitute a network. There is a high degree of cross membership between expert committees of MAFF, the Food and Drink Federation (FDF) and the industry-funded British Nutrition Foundation (BNF). Under these circumstances it seems feasible to argue that a technocratic network does exist because there is a degree of shared expertise in conjunction with loyalties to extra-technical values and policy goals which can largely be explained in terms of career socialisation processes or bureaucratic-administrative goals.

It is not uncommon, however, for technocrats to comprise an element of largely non-technocratic structures, that is, to be strategically placed within a policy community or policy network on the basis of their expertise and loyalty to policy goals. In short, their position is granted on the basis of the resources they can bring to that structure.

How, then, does this characterisation of elites, professionals, technocrats and networks relate to the arguments I forwarded earlier on structure, power and agency?

I have already said that networks, as structures, will display many of the characteristics of policy communities. To this extent, then, all networks will experience mutual adjustment, the uneven distribution of resources, a varying potential for action and will leave monuments to the balance of their forces in terms of standardised expressions of their relationships. In short, networks will have to respond to changing circumstances, will have some interests in them which are more powerful than others, and will be able to create some effect.

Once we have labelled a configuration as a particular type of network (producer, professional etc) it is possible to be more specific about the nature of the relationships that constitute the structure, and about the balance of forces within them. For example, it is obvious that a professionalised network will only contain a certain sort of agent and that these agents will possess certain, scarce, resources. Hence, one would expect that the resources that were shared in common would be far greater than in other networks, although one would still expect some sort of hierarchy. The mutual adjustments between the agents of the network would, therefore, be far smaller. By this I mean that the values, ideology and expressions of the relationships would be particularly strong and, hence, the likelihood of dissent or of large shifts in the resources within the network would be small. Indeed, what is most interesting about networks made up of members with similar characteristics is the fact that shifts in the balance of power within the network actually make very little difference to the effects that the network has on its external environment because the agents are, broadly, political equivalents (non-structural features excepted).

Again, the *processes* within these networks and the *changes* that arise, can be accounted for just as they were with policy communities, that is, in terms of the perceived interests of the members and the distribution of resources either within the network or, more likely, between the network and its external environment.

Professionals, and others holding similar resources cannot, for the purposes of explanation, be seen as occupying only one structure ie. a single professionalised network. Rather, we have to establish where this is appropriate and where it is necessary to plot more precisely the communities and networks of which professionals/elites/technocrats are a part or which affect them.

In terms of this case study, this characterisation fits. What happened within the NHS in response to the evidence on diet and heart disease is very consistent and suggests, because of its uniformity, that the term professionalised network is appropriate. Where professionals were powerful, they responded positively and consistently to the medical evidence. They could do this, in part at least, because of their positions on the policy communities which controlled sub-national decision making.

Other policy communities exist at national level, in, for example, the Nutrition, Preventive Medicine and Coronary Heart Disease Divisions of the DoH. These also have a professional input, as do the expert committees attached to the DoH. In both these instances, it is possible to see that these are serviced by other networks which form around particular aspects of policy. Increasingly, however, as these networks intrude into central government, the rules of the game or the terms of reference become set not by the professionals themselves, as is the case in their "home" network, but by the wider political considerations of governments more generally.

Conclusion

This Chapter has attempted to clarify the meanings of the concepts which this study will use for its theoretical explanations. It has also begun the process of applying these concepts to the interests that can be identified within the policy area under consideration. We have seen how resources can shift from one interest to another through time and how the normal work of political relationships can create expressions of that work.

Policy communities and networks are descriptions of particular parts of structures which have decision making functions and which attempt to control other parts of the structure. However, because they are still structures, much of what applies to communities also applies to networks.

In short, we should expect all political relationships to be under constant pressure to modify their positions because they have to respond to the changing circumstances in which they find themselves. This is why no policy has ever solved a problem once and for all - things change. Networks and communities are types of political relationship which deal with these problems. My argument has been that some networks are more flexible than others, that is, policy communities are quite rigid, inflexible means of decision making. If I am right, then, by implication, the ability of a policy community to take on board new ideas is going to be limited. Such a policy community would much rather live with the problem than change the policies it is attached to. Such a characterisation can explain 1. why change might be necessary in the first place, and 2. why a policy community might not want to change. We will be able to test this once we have seen what the response of successive governments has been to the dietary change debate.

Finally, I have argued that it is sensible, for the sake of precision, to concede that communities can co-exist with networks within the same policy area, so that we can account for the networks which service policy communities, and the responsibilities which are delegated to these networks by policy communities. Again, it will be necessary to be clear on exactly what sort of network we are referring to, whether, for example, it is elite, technocratic, professionalised etc. The differences between these may be of explanatory importance.

This provides the framework within which it is possible to characterise the primary interests within the food and health policy area. On the one hand there are the relationships that exist within and around MAFF, with a dominant policy community, a series of sub-sectors and issue related networks permeated by technocrats and producer interests. On the other hand, there are policy communities within the DoH around their Units (which do not appear to be particularly important for our purposes) and an extended professionalised network within the NHS. In addition, there are elites which feed into central decision making processes in an advisory capacity. The links between these two policy areas are fairly tenuous in structural terms, and appear to be largely informal. As such, the policy areas have developed as discrete networks operating more or less independently of each other.

3 Dietary Change: The Evidence

Dietary change is a very controversial political issue. One reason for this is that very large shifts in consumption patterns will have an equally large effect on agricultural and food processing industries. Consequently, governments and industry need to be assured that the evidence which relates diet to health problems is actually valid.

This chapter does not try to establish whether the evidence relating diet to heart disease is valid or not, primarily because the author is not qualified to judge all the available evidence. Nevertheless, a chapter on the evidence is important. If professionals agree on the causes and the consequences of certain health problems then this is a politically important feature of the politics of dietary change. If professionals make recommendations on how to reduce heart disease, this too is important. Similarly, if governments accept the causal relationship as valid (regardless of whether it turns out to be so in the end) then this will make a difference to any policies which are forthcoming. So, the job of this chapter is less to evaluate the evidence itself, than to show (1) that heart disease is a problem, (2) that professionals do agree that it is related to diet, and (3) what professionals have recommended governments do about the problem.

Diet and Coronary Heart Disease (CHD) displays many, if not all, of the characteristics associated with dietary change in general. It is typical in the disputes over the validity of the scientific evidence, the economic consequences of dietary change, who should promote change (professionals or governments) and how far the state should act on behalf of the individual. In all these senses the evidence and the implications of diet and heart disease illustrate much broader features of the food and health policy area.

Heart Disease : The Evidence

The evidence linking diet to the incidence of CHD has been very controversial and has generated a great deal of debate within the medical profession and between other interested parties such as food manufacturers, farmers and consumer groups. Scientifically, the problem has revolved around the burden of proof and the methodological tools available to provide it. Politically, the discussion has been rather less scientific and has centred, either explicitly or implicitly, on the political and economic implications of accepting the relationship and the recommendations which invariably accompany it.

There are three reasons for looking at the scientific evidence. The first is simply that it demonstrates one of the central themes of this study, namely, that changes in scientific orthodoxy can be a prolonged and controversial affair which can have political consequences. Secondly, it highlights the fact that such change often comes from professional elites rather than the mass of practising professionals - this is an important empirical and theoretical point. Thirdly, and perhaps most importantly, the exercise will provide part of the basis for arguing that CHD is a problem in Britain (the other part will come in the following section). It will also provide part of the necessary background information for evaluating and presenting the implications for policies dealing to diet and health.

Epidemiological evidence has suggested that there are certain diseases which are far more prevalent in industrialised societies and in other, pre-industrial ones. Hence the expression, "diseases of affluence".[1] The implication is that these diseases have an environmental origin:

---

1 The expression "diseases of affluence" is a misleading one. It refers to diseases in affluent societies as opposed to non-affluent societies. Within affluent societies, however, these diseases are generally inversely related to class.

...many of these diseases are rare or virtually unknown
in societies which in all material ways seem to be far
less fortunate, and where, in general, people seem far
more prone to disease (Tudge;1983,p32).

This is true of CHD (See - WHO;1982). The process of identifying the
particular aspects of industrialised societies responsible for these incidence
levels began in the late 1950's and early in the 1960's with a number of
studies, the most famous of which was the Framingham Study
(McNair;1988). This, and other studies, identified four major risk factors
which were manipulable and believed to increase an individuals risk of
contracting heart disease - smoking, the level of cholesterol in the blood,
high blood pressure and lack of exercise. Age sex and family history were
also important risk factors but, of course, they cannot be manipulated. The
general principle behind identifying the prevalence of risk factors within
populations and individuals is simply that the more of them there are, the
greater the likelihood of CHD. Because they are more prevalent in
industrialised societies CHD is more common.

However, this still leaves a number of central questions unanswered.
Firstly, which aspect of diet causes CHD, and secondly, does it necessarily
follow that by modifying the risk factor[s] the risk of CHD is reduced?

The answer to the first question is bio-chemical and has itself been the
subject of some debate (BMA;1986 Royal College;1976). The level of
cholesterol in the blood is raised by the consumption of saturated fats. In
the western diet this comes primarily from animal products and hardened
fat the major sources of which are red meat, milk, cheese, margarine and
butter although there is a lot of hidden fat in such things as cakes, biscuits,
pastry and meat products. Saturated fat stimulates the liver to produce
more cholesterol than the body actually needs (the liver creates cholesterol
anyway). Cholesterol then travels in the blood stream and is deposited on
the inside of the arteries - a process known as arterioscleroma. The arteries
are gradually furred up by this process which may eventually restrict the
supply of blood to the heart when the blood clots and hence cause a heart
attack. This process is also implicated in cerebrovascluar disease (ie.
stroke). Collectively, this group of diseases are called cardiovascular
diseases.

The professional debate has centred on the question of whether saturated
fats were causally related to this process and whether   PUFA's
(Polyunsaturated Fatty Acids) were protective in any way. There now

42

seems to be broad agreement that a causal relationship does exist and that changing the ratio of saturated to unpolyunsaturated fat in the diet (in favour of the latter) would have health benefits.

The answer to the second question (would modifying risk factors help?) is less straightforward. The correlation between the consumption of saturated fat and the incidence of heart disease is strong between populations, that is, when comparing bushmen and Glaswegians. Within populations, however, the variations between individuals appears to produce less convincing results. As a result, modifying risk factors, eg. reducing the cholesterol in any given individual, may not prevent heart disease, although modifying the intake of saturated fat in the whole population should reduce everybodies risk. It is on this point that there has been considerable debate because it implies that to counter CHD whole populations should modify their risk factors. Some elite professionals appear to be more willing to give this advice than others who have demanded proof that the advice is valid. Ideally, this proof would take the form of a clinical trial which could monitor groups who are having their risk factors modified, against those who are not. However, there are methodological and financial problems with this approach. Financially,these trials are very expensive:

> Further conclusive evidence leading to proof on the question of diet and coronary heart disease is most unlikely to come within the next ten years, if at all. In the United States it was calculated that a dietary trial large enough to provide a conclusive answer would have cost in 1969 between 250 and 500 million dollars, and hence it was not carried out (Ball and Turner;1974,p740).

The methodological problems have been highlighted by Tudge:

> Suppose, for example, that our hypothetical mega-scientist wanted to test the idea that excessive fat intake leads to coronary heart disease. The obvious way to go about this would be to keep two colonies of laboratory humans, one fed a high fat, the other a low fat diet...human beings are extremely variable in their response to fat...[so]   he would have to have large colonies.
> Another possibility, well worth investigating, is that

43

changes in the arteries that lead to coronary heart
disease may begin early in life. To test this...our tire-
less super-scientist would have to maintain his colonies
of several thousand individuals through their entire lives
(Tudge;1983,p32-33).

Given that this is neither possible or desirable,another way of testing the
hypothesis that CHD is positively correlated to saturated fat intake is to
conduct intervention trials. These trials intervene in the sense that they
counsel, inform and educate sample populations to see if this affects their
rate of heart disease. Examples of such trials are the Multiple Risk Factor
Intervention Trial (MRFIT) in the USA (Multiple;1981) and the North
Karelia Project (Finland) (Puska et al;1981). These generally took place in
the 1970's and are the trials which followed those which identified the risk
factors (Farchi;1984,p219-224). Again, however, proof was elusive. In
the MRFIT and North Karelia studies for example, the incidence of heart
disease did fall in the intervention group, but it also fell in the control group
as well, although not by as much. The problem is whether the CHD rate
was falling of its own accord or whether intervention was necessary to
induce such a fall.

The explanation for these results is simply that in order to obtain a
control group which was similar to the intervention group, both groups (in
both studies) were geographically close to each other. Because of this, and
because of the nature of the intervention which was difficult to confine to
one particular part of the community, the control group picked up on the
advice and counselling and acted accordingly.

Similarly, a study in Oslo (Preventive Medicine;1985) used a sample of
middle aged men (those believed to be most at risk) and had promising
results in terms of reducing both mortality and morbidity by modifying
smoking and eating habits. This does not automatically imply, however,
that similar strategies would be successful across complete populations.

Despite the methodological objections, in those countries where health
professionals have been willing to act without absolute proof, the rate of
heart disease has fallen dramatically. In the USA and Australia, for
example, the incidence of heart disease fell by 30% between 1970 and
1980. In Canada, Belgium and Japan it has fallen by 20% (Nursing
Times;1987,p24-26).

By the early 1980's a consensus was clearly evident among the majority
of professional elite organisations. This confirmed the correlation between
diet and heart disease largely, it appears, because there was deemed to be

sufficient evidence pointing in the same direction and few substantial or inexplicable objections to the central thesis:

> The panel...has acknowledged that the evidence falls short of proof. Nevertheless, if changes in diet occur in the directions recommended, benefits to health are likely (DHSS;1984,p1).
> ...now seems an appropriate time for energetic action based on the balance of probabilities (Royal College;1976,p218).
> The scientific evidence...does not amount to certain proof but it is reasonable grounds for energetic action (Interdisciplinary;1984,p2).

Despite these reservations, "consensus" is now the word being used:

> The statements from the EAS (European Arterio-sclerosis Society) and the BCS (British Cardiac Society)...reflects a medical consensus, both in the United Kingdom and across the whole of Europe, that coronary heart disease rates...should be reduced by...reducing smoking, reducing dietary fat and increas-ing exercise in the population (Lancet;1987,p601-602).

> ...this is an overwhelming professional consensus on action (J o Royal College;1985,p59-60).

There still remains the question of which strategy would be most likely to reduce the incidence of CHD. Again, there has been disagreement, this time between those who favour taking the "population approach", and those who want to concentrate on identifying those at high risk - the "at risk" approach. The population approach asserts that if everyone modifies their risk factors then the incidence of CHD will fall. The "at risk" approach, however, argues that strategies should concentrate only on those who are most likely to contract the disease. The diagram below (Figure 3.0) suggests that simply using the at risk approach will not be sufficient to reduce CHD significantly.

Figure 3.0 confirms that the greater a persons level of blood cholesterol, the greater their chances of having CHD. But it also shows that those who are at high risk are only a small proportion of the population and, in absolute terms, constitute a smaller of total deaths (about 30%). A far higher proportion of deaths come from the category which has a medium risk, simply because there are so many more people in this category. To some extent both approaches have been accepted as valid as it is now believed that a population strategy should be supplemented by the vigorous identification of those most at risk. In dietary terms the target which now seems to be consensual is that fat intake should not provide more than 35% of a persons total calories (DHSS;1984,p5)

Fig. 3. The relationship between a population distribution of serum cholesterol concentration, an estimate of the rise of death from coronary heart disease at each level of cholesterol concentration and an estimate of the number of deaths attributable to cholesterol concentrations above the minimum band shown. Source: HEC:1983,p17.

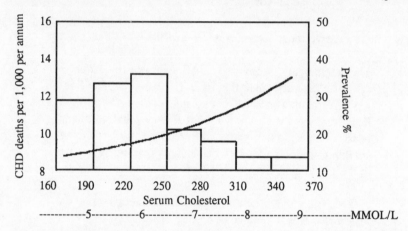

It is not difficult to see the scientific, methodological and "strategy" problems which diet and CHD presents. Regardless of what we may think about the validity of the evidence itself, the controversy and its effects are politically important. The broad agreement which has emerged during the 1980's suggests that while discussion will continue over how much CHD can be explained by diet, there are few professionals (elite or otherwise) who would deny that a causal relationship exists and that there are strategies available to prevent its worst effects. For our purposes, this is all we need to know.

Heart Disease in Britain

As an industrialised country, Britain is as prone to "diseases of affluence" as any other. Fat consumption has risen steadily since the beginning of the century and dropped in the mid-1970's before levelling off somewhere between 38-42% of total calories. Carbohydrates (starches and sugars) have been falling, although sugar has only fallen since the 1960's. Protein has remained fairly static and total energy has risen despite the fact that people tend to lead more sedentary lives.

It is not difficult to demonstrate the prevalence of CHD in Britain. In 1978, for example, 106,000 men and nearly 79,000 women died from the disease, in 1984 the total figure was 175,000 (Smith and Jacobson;1988,p29); that amounts to approximately one every three or four minutes (DHSS;1981,p24). As a proportion of total deaths, heart disease is the biggest single cause for both men and women.

Table 3.0. Proportion of all deaths from the given causes (1982). England and Wales.

	Males	Females
Coronary Heart Disease	31%	23%
Cerebrovascular Disease	9%	15%
Cancers	24%	21%
All Other causes	36%	41%

Source: Office of Population and Censuses Surveys in DHSS;1984,p14

There has been a downward trend in absolute CHD mortality since the mid-1960's although as a proportion of all deaths it has been rising during this period. This cannot be explained in terms of the increase in life expectancy (ie. the longer you live the more likely you are to contract heart disease) because those most at risk are middle aged men, and the average blood cholesterol level does not increase significantly for this category between the ages of 44 and 59.

So, while an older population might be expected to contract more heart disease this cannot account for the increasing incidence in young middle age. In short, this means: "60% of middle aged men in this country have a twofold or greater risk of coronary heart disease from their blood cholesterol level alone (Shaper;1989,p12)". This level was found to be 20% in excess of the level which the WHO thought constituted a low risk.

The human consequences of heart disease are therefore enormous. With something approaching one death in three resulting from heart disease there are few families that are not directly affected. The further tragedy is that many "die young" from the disease. One quarter of deaths from CHD occur before the age of 65. This amounts to 250,000 years of potential life lost

(OHE;1982,p51).

But the costs of CHD can be measured in other ways as well. The Office of Health Economics, for example, calculated the financial cost to the NHS of heart disease:

Table 3.1. Estimated Cost of Medical Care for CHD in 1981, England and Wales.

	Cost in £m.
Approx' 2.5m In-Patient Days	153.8
Out-Patients	6.6
Pharmaceuticals (18.2m Prescriptions)	84.5
General Medical Services	9.9
Total Cost	254.8

Source: OHE Estimates. (OHE;1982,p46). [2]

In addition there were 26 million working days lost because of CHD in 1979/80 with all the consequent costs in terms of lost production and National Insurance Fund Payments (£115m) (OHE;1982,p51).

But CHD is also a class-related disease. While in the past it was believed that middle class, hypertensive executives were most prone to CHD the reality is that CHD, as with most of the other major causes of death, is inversely related to social class (Rose et al;1977,p105-9). Similarly, CHD rates are the highest in areas which have traditionally been seen as predominantly working class; South Wales, the North East, Northern Ireland and Scotland (DHSS;1981,p26).

Table 3.2. Standardised Mortality Ratios for Coronary Heart Disease and all causes by Social Class, England and Wales (1972).

Social Class	CHD	All Causes
I	88	77
II	91	81
III non-manual	114	99
III manual	107	106
IV	108	114
V	111	137

Source: Office of Population, Censuses and Surveys, in, National Forum:1988,p36.[3]

---

2 The figure given by the OHE (£254.8m) is approximately half that estimated by the National Audit Office (NAO) in 1989. I have given the OHE table because it gives the distribution of costs and the NAO do not.

3 Smith and Jacobson (1988) provide more recent figures but this table specifies CHD

The relationship between CHD and class is not quite as pronounced as it is for "all causes" because Social Class III (non-manual) does not conform to the expected pattern. Nevertheless, with this exception the relationship is clear and consistent. The apparent predisposition of lower socio-economic groups to CHD can be explained through a combination of factors. Firstly, as the Black Report highlighted, working people are less likely to make the best use of the health service or, more importantly, to use the preventive services (Townsend and Davidson;1982,p81). Equally, they are more likely to smoke (an important risk factor) and have diets which are generally higher in saturated fats.

Similarly, it has been argued that those on state support are unlikely to have an income which is sufficient to buy an adequate diet (Walker and Church; 1978). A study of Manchester's poor found:

> A disturbingly high number of people are not eating because of lack of money.
> Amongst all those on low incomes unemployed people are the hardest hit, for example missing meals, not having enough money to buy food, and cutting back on food when short of cash.
> Despite the high level of general concern about their food, lack of money restricted peoples means to eat well (Lang et al;1984, p41).

Other factors which may effect CHD, such as chronic stress, have also been seen as widespread in working class communities (Farrent and Russell;1985,p20). Lower socio-economic groups have to contend with all the usual risk factors while being short on the income and information which would allow some amelioration of those factors.

Perhaps the single most telling testimony to the scale of Britain's CHD problem comes from comparing the incidence of CHD in Britain to the rates in other industrialised countries.

As it stands Table 3.3 indicates that Britain has one of the worst rates of CHD in the industrialised world which, in essence, means that if CHD is a problem of industrialised societies it is a particularly large problem in Britain.

---

deaths. Since 1972, the inverse relationship between social class and premature death has, if anything, become stronger.

Table 3.3. Death rates for coronary heart disease (ICD 410-414) for the fourteen highest ranking countries in 1978 (age standardized rates/100,000; 35-74 year age group).

Males   Female

Males		Female	
Finland	664	Scotland	256
Scotland	656	Northern Ireland	233
Northern Ireland	653	Israel	207
Ireland	542	Ireland	200
England and Wales	533	New Zealand	196
NewZealand	529	USA	187
USA	506	Australia	186
Australia	499	Finland	177
Canada	457	England and Wales	173
Denmark	443	Hungary	168
Sweden	436	Bulgaria	162
Hungary	420	Canada	155
Norway	414	Denmark	141
Israel	395	Sweden	132

Source: DHSS; 1984.p16

In fact, Britain's comparative position is worse than the table suggests.Since these figures were compiled many of the countries mentioned have experienced rapidly falling rates of CHD. Notable amon;st these are Finland, Israel, the USA, Australia, New Zealand and Canada (BMJ;1987). Britain on the other hand has declined very little in comparison and as a result the comparative incidence of CHD is getting worse.

This is not to say that deaths from CHD in Britain are not falling, nor does it imply that saturated fat consumption has not fallen during the 1980's. The evidence suggests that there has been an improvement in both these indecies, but it also suggests (1) Britain's problem remains large and (2) other countries which started from a much lower base have experienced more success in reducing CHD than Britain. Perhaps other countries are doing something Britain is not?

Norway and the United States

The most interesting thing to come out of a look at the strategies of other countries is not the models they produce, but the explanations that can be found for the differences in strategies across countries. It seems clear that in the two examples given here these differences owe a great deal to the cultural and institutional differences their political systems display.

Norway provides an example of an interventionist state which has had a social-democratic consensus for much of the post war period. This consensus is reflected not only in the role of the state, but also in the institutional arrangements for formulating and implementing policy. The Norwegian parliament is comparatively weak, which is, perhaps, to be expected where adversarial politics is uncommon and a great deal of policy is made in sub-central agencies. Within these agencies interests are incorporated into the policy making process through their representative organisations. As Olsen observes:

> ...integrated participation occurs more frequently in the Scandinavian countries than in Great Britain and much more frequently than in the United States (Olsen; 1983,p166).

Many of these agencies are dominated by economic and labour interests and it appears that the system works particularly well in reducing conflict between the two sides of industry. It should also be noted that farming, food manufacturing and fishing groups are also given access to these agencies. As a consequence there is: "...a broad acceptance of integrated participation in Norwegian policy making (Olsen;1983,p177)".

Thus, cooption is a central feature of policy making in Norway which suggests not only an extended role for the state in, for example, agricultural subsidies but also a broad consensus that this is desirable. Consequently, there are also the institutional mechanisms available to facilitate the generation of those policies. This facility can, as we shall see, extend across policy boundaries. The image that is created, therefore, is of a homogeneous political structure which relies very much upon central and sub-central government agencies for the resolution of conflict and the development of policy. Furthermore, the impression is given that the institutional mechanisms necessary to deliver those policies are available and, in terms of economic growth at least, have been successful (Ringen;1979).

Norway has experienced the shifts in consumption patterns which characterise industrialised societies - a marked reduction in fruit and vegetable consumption and increases in meat and dairy products in the past 50 years (Winikoff;1977,p552). It also has the high rates of cardiovascular diseases that might be expected: "In Norway, over one half of all deaths occur as a result of cardiovascular diseases" (Winikoff;1977,p552), an increase of 280 and 180% for men and women respectively over the previous 20 years (Ringen;1977,p37).

Unlike many other western countries, however, Norway has a history of taking its national and international responsibilities for food very seriously. It was, for example, alone in complying with the recommendations of the World Food Conference of 1974 to develop domestic policies with the third world in mind (Ringen;1979,p33).

What is perhaps most remarkable, however, is the Norwegian "Food and Nutrition Policy". This policy is unique to the extent that it attempts to integrate a number of food and nutrition goals into a single policy. These fall into four categories:

1. To stimulate the consumption of healthy foodstuffs;
2. To develop guidelines for food production in accordance with the recommendations of the World Food Council;
3. To increase self-sufficiency;
4. To strengthen rural districts and maintain their living standards (Ringen;1977,p550).

Many of these initiatives are building on existing political commitments. The Norwegian state already accepted responsibility for equalising the pay of farm workers and industrial workers and there have previously been attempts to increase domestic food production. Hence, many of the institutional mechanisms of, for example, consultation, negotiation and implementation, already existed.

The reduction of CHD was highlighted as an objective of the broader policy, it was argued that fat should not contribute more than 35% of total calories, and preferably no more than 30%. As Ringen argues:

> The policy is also unique in the context of the traditional
> role of government in western societies. It is based on a
> professionally determined optimum diet (Ringen;1979,
> p33).

The Norwegian Board of Health had made strong recommendations on heart disease and diet in 1972 (BMJ;1972,p539). Such deference to professional opinion has led the Norwegian government to commit itself to utilising those mechanisms which are available to it to achieve its nutritional goals. These mechanisms are varied and include the restructuring of agricultural subsidies to encourage both the production and consumption of healthier foods; the strict surveillance of food advertising and of educational material distributed in schools; education within schools about both good nutritional practice and the system of food supply; the funding of research by the government into, for example, the development of fish products (as opposed to meat products) and the provision of funds for advertising, health education and the dissemination of information (Royal Norwegian; 1981,p10-11).

While many of these policy objectives exist in other countries (they are not entirely absent even in Britain) what is striking about the Norwegian example is (1) that these various goals all exist within one policy and (2) that it is the goals that take precedence over procedural or administrative considerations of implementation. Thus, the policy constitutes not only the goals themselves, but also the creation and utilisation of administrative facilities to secure its objectives.

> Because of the comprehensive nature of the policy, the responsibilities for its implementation will have to be divided among [eight] different ministries .....An interministerial body will be established to coordinate these responsibilities. The National Nutrition Council (established in 1946) will be reorganized, and an office of nutrition will be established in the Ministry of Social Affairs (Ringen;1979,p39).

Again, this represents a particular conception of what responsibilities the state should take in conjunction with a willingness to utilise and expand the existing institutional arrangements for implementation.

While the political motivations for the policy are diverse because there is more than one goal to the policy, it is particularly interesting that a policy which originally had a purely agricultural focus was able to accommodate professional advice and adapt accordingly. The elevation of the principles of public health to the status of a serious policy objective reflects both the ideological predisposition of successive Norwegian governments to intervene in the functioning of the market when it believes this is necessary, and also the historical interest that the state has taken in food and nutrition. Importantly, however, this type of approach has been developed in a consensual political environment, where there are mechanisms available for the incorporation of genuine interests. As such, the system is responsive and it can operate with the cooperation of economic interests because they are part of the decision making processes themselves. Similarly, the fact that health professionals enjoy similar integration means that there is political access. Health professionals do not compete for access into these centres as is the case in the US or Britain, but rather, are utilised by the state to resolve politically and professionally defined problems. So, even though health professionals may be the motor of dietary change, their work is mediated through a paternalistic and interventionist state apparatus which assumes responsibility for dietary goals. This is not to say that Norway is without its problems. It would be wrong to suggest that conflicts do not arise; it is known for example, that consumer interests and those of less powerful groups find it much more difficult to influence policy than industry and the labour unions. My argument is not that Norway is a social democratic paradise, but rather, that it does have an active and involved state apparatus which affords opportunities for organised participation.

In the United States, institutional arrangements and state responsibilities are quite different. Unlike Norway, the United States has a federal system of government in which federal (national) government is comparatively weak. Equally, the ideological orientation is far less interventionist in general and this is reflected in the institutional arrangements of central government and the responsibilities it assumes. Health care provides a good example of this.

In contrast to most western countries, the United States does not have a comprehensive system of health insurance and, until recently, did not have a federal department committed solely to health issues. While there existed departments of agriculture, for example, which also enjoyed coordinating committees with other departments, policies on health developed in an ad hoc and largely uncoordinated way (Lee;1979). The federalist structure of government meant that central government tended to fund state level initiatives in, for example, child welfare, research and planning in an attempt to equalise health care throughout the United States but these policies developed incrementally and almost by default as a result of pressures from interest groups. Federal government became responsible for paying approximately half of health care costs through, for example, medical insurance to the aged and very poor, welfare and hospital building, while leaving a generally dynamic and largely unfettered health profession.

Indeed, through the American Medical Association, the profession is keen to retain its independence from government as far as possible (Ward;1979) because it sees health as a market like most others, and hence, federal and state interference is not appreciated.

While it would be wrong to suggest that central government is ineffective, there are clearly differences between the roles of the state in Norway and the United States. At the federal (central) level, there is less formal cooption of organisations in the United States, and this applies particularly to health and welfare groups. As Olsen noted (1983,p173), even economic interests tend to work through multinational companies rather than peak organisations - a trend which is increasingly obvious in Britain as well. Even though there is now a Department of Health and Human Services, historically, the ideological predisposition of the state and its administrative arrangements have militated against comprehensive and integrated policies across policy boundaries. Lastly, in terms of health professionals, there appears to be an institutionalised separation of the state and professionals, with the latter acting in large part as simply "another" - albeit very powerful - group and having little formal incorporation into decision making processes.

So, there are some notable differences between the political systems of Norway and the United States. Crucially, it appears as though in the US the ability and willingness of central government to coopt, integrate and coordinate interests is very limited whereas in Norway this is an accepted part of political life. Interestingly, however, each preserves its commitment to liberal-democratic values and to the freedom of the market place, but interprets the states' responsibilities in a different way.

Winikoff (1977) makes some telling comparisons between the Norwegian and United States' governments attitudes to nutrition policies. She argues very strongly that in the United States the federal government has been loathe to take substantive steps to formulate a national policy which would reflect the advice of professionals and experts:

> ...in contrast to Norway's, the American dietary goals
> are only weakly linked to policy. The logical process
> whereby necessity for dietary change leads to the
> formation of policy to change the food system is not
> addressed here (Winikoff;1977,p553).

She further argues that while the US government does, in reality, intervene in the food supply through such things as food stamps, farm subsidies, taxation and welfare provision, none of these have been utilised to further the nutritional well-being of the population. Even though one half of all deaths in the United States were caused by cardiovascular disease in 1972, central government had done little to counteract this; the Senate Select Committee on Nutrition and Human Needs was the only source of guidance on this issue:

> Interestingly, in contrast to Norway where the proposals [for dietary change] arose from the central circle of government power, this task was not undertaken by official policymaking agencies of the executive branch (Winikoff;1977,p553).

A Senate Select Committee report (the McGovern Report;1977) made recommendations about food labelling, research and education but did not comment on the mechanisms and priorities that might best facilitate dietary changes. This is entirely consistent with the characterisation of US policy in the health-welfare field given above - there are official exhortations but the mechanisms to translate these into comprehensive policies are simply not available. This does not necessarily imply that change is impossible, but rather, that if there is change, then it is unlikely to come about because of central political agencies.

Surprisingly, perhaps, the fall in the rate of heart disease in the United States has been very large over the past 25 years - a decline of about 30%. At first sight this would appear to contradict Winikoff's argument that the US government was not doing enough in terms of promoting dietary change. A report by the US Department of Agriculture in 1976 argued that nearly half the respondents to a survey it conducted said that they had changed their diet for health reasons (The New England;1985), and this too would appear to contradict Winikoff.

In fact, it is not the government that is responsible for this reduction, it is health professionals:

> Since 1959, experts have repeatedly advised American physicians, other public health professionals, policy-makers and the public on the major risk factors [of coronary heart disease](The New England;1985, p1053-1055).

The process of change actually began earlier with a certain Dr. Jollife and the Anti-Coronary Club of New York in 1956. He advocated a "prudent diet" which included a reduction in saturated fat consumption. In 1957 the American Heart Association began to argue that diet was, in part, to blame for the prevalence of heart disease and in 1961 it started to promote the prudent diet for those who were most at risk of CHD. By 1965, this advice was extended to the whole population, and in 1968, there was specific and quantified advice on fat consumption (Turner;1983b,pp10-11).[4] The burden of scientific proof does not seem to have afflicted the US medical profession to the extent that it has the British. It seems clear that, as Turner (1983) argues, in the US: "...leadership of the dietary campaign came from the medical profession (Turner;1983a,p42)".

Since Winikoff wrote, the official position on health promotion has changed in the United States. Notably, the US has fulfilled its obligations under the World Health Organisation's Alma Mata declaration (to which Britain was a signatory) that it would set measurable health goals to be achieved by the year 2000. Such a commitment is in line with the WHO's "Health for All by the Year 2000" campaign (Interdisciplinary;1984,pp6-7).

Thus we get the impression of a fragmented political response to the problem of dietary change in the United States. Again professionals are the motor for change, but in the US the professionals appear to act autonomously and have achieved reductions in CHD without large scale active involvement from the state.

The differences in approach adopted by Norway and the United States can be explained by a number of different factors. It seems clear, for example, that the ideological predisposition of the state is important to the extent that it partly determines what the state believes its responsibilities are. In turn, this will affect the type of administrative-institutional framework that exists. Thus, Norway has a comprehensive system of sub-central agencies to facilitate the cooption of organisations, while in the United States, less formal and more ad hoc arrangements exist. On this basis, it is ideologically and institutionally more likely that the state in Norway should be active in promoting dietary change because many of the necessary political structures and relationships already exist.

These arrangements also bring with them a certain division of responsibility between the state and health professionals. In the United States neither the federal nor the state governments take the degree of responsibility for health care provision that is evident in Britain nor do they operate a scheme of comprehensive health insurance as in Norway.

---

4 By way of contrast, this type of advice was not seen in Britain until 1983.

Because of this, and the heterogeneous nature of the health care delivery system, the profession is more dynamic and prone to experiment. While a great part of research funding comes from federal government, it is nevertheless true that the American profession appears to operate far more independently of central government than is the case in Norway. Consequently, initiatives can be taken and can be applied in the absence of state support. This is consistent with Hollingsworth's argument that unitary and centralised systems tend to be less innovative than those which are diversified (Hollingsworth;1986). Given this, it is perhaps unsurprising that in the US the role of health professionals has been enhanced, and the role of the state minimal.

However, it does not follow that where there is less government intervention in health provision there is a more effective health service. Nor does it mean that Winikoff was wrong to suggest that the US government was not taking its responsibilities seriously enough. A closer look at the US decline in the rate of heart disease shows that it has fallen unevenly across class boundaries. While the fall has been some 38% among the middle class, within the working class it has been only 16% (The New England;1985,pp1053-1055). In other words, while health professionals may accomplish many things on their own they cannot instigate a comprehensive policy which will reach those most affected by the disease. If success is to spread beyond these groups then some sort of state intervention in product control (labelling, compositional standards, advertising) and health education would appear necessary.

Nevertheless, Norway and the United States are often held to represent examples of what can be achieved both politically and professionally. Both their approaches are interesting because they represent two distinct methods of tackling the same problem with success, but with historical and ideological variations expressed in the separation of the responsibilities allocated within their social and political systems. The potential for success, in terms of the ability to reduce heart disease across class boundaries in particular is probably greater in Norway because there is a far more comprehensive range of resources that can be applied. In short then, when looking at how countries deal with problems such as these, you would expect to find some correlation between the type of responsibilities they have taken in the past, and the means that are available to solve the problem.

In both these cases action has come far earlier than it has in Britain. Even though the medical consensus on heart disease did not emerge until the late 1970's, many professional organisations and Departments of Health had issued recommendations to the general public in the absence of absolute proof or consensus. Cannon (1987b) documents 65 reports published between 1965 and 1987, all of which comprise what he calls "Universal Agreement on Food and Health"; 20 of these were published between 1965 and 1976 (Cannon;1987b,p29). While this evidence was sufficient to produce profound changes in political and professional thinking in many countries of the industrialised world (Norway, the United States, Australia, New Zealand, Sweden for example) in Britain, where the incidence of heart disease was amongst the highest the politically induced changes were largely imperceptible. Britain, therefore, lags behind those countries with comparable rates of heart disease by about 10 years. This is partly the responsibility of the elite professionals themselves (see Chapter 6), but even when an unequivocal professional message did emerge, it did not have a profound effect on public policy.

Implications for Britain

We have seen what the evidence is to link diet to CHD and we also know that CHD is a major problem in Britain. But is it possible to discern a strategy which professionals believe will reduce CHD? In other words, what policies do they want? Of course it is difficult to aggregate the opinions of a whole profession - inevitably something will be lost in the aggregation. Nevertheless there is a great deal of common ground between them and to illustrate the major points that have been made by health professionals, we will look at four reports; the British Medical Associations' (BMA) *"Diet, Nutrition and Health"* (1986); *"The Prevention of Coronary Heart Disease : Plans for Action"* (which was a report based on a conference-workshop in 1984 organised by the Coronary Prevention Group(CPG); the World Health Organisations' (WHO) *"The Prevention of Coronary Heart Disease"* (1982) and the National Forum for Heart Disease Preventions' *"Coronary Heart Disease Prevention: Action in the UK 1984-1987."* (1988). Through these reports it is possible to find four broad features of policy which seem to be commonly advocated.

A Preventive Strategy

The first and most obvious point to make is that heart disease requires a preventive strategy. The scale of the problem in Britain make a curative response both undesirable and ultimately ineffective; undesirable because

CHD can only be cured once it has struck; ineffective, both because you cannot cure the dead, and because the incidence of CHD will continue to increase without prevention and will ultimately become economically and organisationally unmanageable. The DoH recognises that such a strategy is best, although is less strident in promoting its own role:

> Prevention is better than cure. It is no good waiting until coronary heart disease restricts your activities; heart surgery is expensive and can only help a few (DHSS;1981,p64)

> We consider that the present size of the CHD problem in this country and the small effect of medical and surgical treatment on the mortality rates of CHD justify attempts to prevent the disease we cannot cure (Royal College;1976,p218).

A Strategy for the Population and Those At Risk

Given that most deaths from CHD come from those people who are deemed to be at moderate risk, health professionals have concluded that everyone in the population should modify their saturated fat and total fat intake. Given also that these reductions may not be sufficient for those who are at high risk of CHD, the "at risk" approach of targetting and seeking out those most vulnerable is seen as a necessary supplement to the broader approach. A necessary corollary to this is that there should be:

A National Policy and Local Level Initiatives

The consensus of opinion appears to be that any country with a CHD problem needs a national policy:

> Effective population prevention of CHD can only come about through national policy, planning, development and commitment (WHO;1982,p36)
> There is an urgent need for the British government.....to formulate national policies and programmes for health promotion and disease prevention (Interdisciplinary;1984,p7)

Some of the reasons for this are given below, but some of them can be given here. To begin with, a national policy, properly defined, provides two things. One is a set of targets or goals that can be used both to direct policies (eg. to base advice and information on) and to measure the success of the efforts that have been made. There is broad agreement that the targets in Britain should be that total fat should not constitute more than 35% of total calories, and that saturated fat should be below 15% of total calories. At the moment, the figures are 42% and 20% respectively.

A national policy also designates the means to accomplish these targets. These means will necessarily have a national and a local component. At national level, health professionals have argued that governments can crucially affect the likely success of anti-coronary strategies through creating, or manipulating, the political and economic environment in which the strategies operate. However, it is also believed that community level action is necessary. This is particularly true of the WHO and Canterbury reports, which both stress that effective strategies will only come about at this level:

> Neighbourhood health strategies and programmes are crucial to grass-roots progress. There is a need for special initiatives to develop or to use existing neighbourhood groups to integrate both professional and community effort (Interdisciplinary;1984,p22).

The crux of this argument is that there exists the need for a "mobilisation" of resources at this level which is seen to involve the National Health Service, Local Authorities and the education system as well.

These two different levels of approach are not independent of each other because national decisions can constrain and facilitate local initiatives. So, health professionals believe central agencies should provide the means, where necessary, to allow the local agencies to comply with the national plan. The examples which are given usually include ear-marking funds for the NHS, providing information material to NHS staff, or supplying a platform for prevention through national campaigns.

The National Plan should be Consistent

A national plan to reduce the incidence of heart disease is, by definition, going to involve both a multi-factoral approach to the problem of heart disease and is going to affect a number of different policy areas as a consequence. The experiences of other countries have shown that for the policy to work to its full potential and, in particular, for it to have a reasonable chance of circumventing socio-ecomonic obstacles, these diverse policy areas should consistently support efforts to reduce heart disease. Sweden, for example, failed to reduce their rates of heart disease as quickly as expected partly because they had also failed to remove subsidies on high fat agricultural products. Fat consumption increased, after an initial fall of 2%, because farmers were given increased subsidies on beef, butter, pork and cheese (Blythe;1976,p279:Welin;1983,pp1087-1089). But prevention can also be a financially worthwhile exercise - Switzerland is an example. It has been argued (Gutzwiller;1987) that by having a heart disease prevention strategy the Swiss have saved twice the cost of the prevention programme through the savings they have made in treating the disease. The point, therefore, is twofold. Firstly, the incidence of heart disease is affected by policies in other policy areas, and secondly, prevention can be a financially consistent strategy to adopt.

This principle has led health professionals to identify a number of areas which offer either facilities for prevention or constraints upon it. Consistency would need to account for both of these, that is, taking opportunities and removing, where possible, obstacles. For example, the re-structuring of agricultural support subsidies (National Forum;1988,pp69-70: Interdisciplinary;1984,p14), the use of the education and health system to inform the emerging adults (WHO;1982,p36: Interdisciplinary;1984,p44), nutritional and compositional labelling (DHSS;1984,p12: Interdisciplinary; 1984,p18: Royal College;1976,p216), and providing consumers with food which corresponds to the new knowledge on health. (DHSS;1984,p12; Interdisciplinary;1984,p15).

But consistency in this context can also mean *coordination* and the need to coordinate anti-coronary policies has been a feature of successive national and international reports:

> A key task...is one of ensuring that the health implications of governmental and industrial actions are clearly recognised before decisions which might have an adverse effect on the risks for coronary heart disease are taken (Interdisciplinary;1984,p5).

There have been various suggestions as to how this might be done; a health seat on NEDDY, a National Nutrition Council, inter-departmental committees, using the Select Committee on Agriculture to monitor progress, a cabinet coordinating committee etc. The essence of all these proposals is that health should be a greater determining factor in public policy in general and that heart disease warrants particular attention.

These, then, are the four broad categories into which professional recommendations fall. Much detail has of necessity been omitted, and some of the more important of these will surface at other times. I have drawn attention to those things which are seen as the most important by health professionals (primarily the elites) and which will have some direct bearing on the actions of governments. From our point of view the exercise was necessary for two reasons. Firstly because the effect professions have on policy can only be assessed if we know what they wanted in the first place. Secondly, when we look at the historical development of policies on food and health, it is useful to be able to contrast these with the policies which are now being proposed by health professionals.

Conclusion

What are the major conclusions that can be drawn at this stage? The first is that there is a broad agreement amongst professionals about the relationship between diet and heart disease. A second conclusion is that the professional view cannot be seen as radical in any meaningful sense of the word. I mentioned earlier that socio-economic variables affect the likelihood of CHD and yet the strategy does not include, for example, the re-distribution of wealth. Neither does it demand the abolition of chemical fertilisers or for taxing foods seen to be unhealthy in some way. Equally, the recommendations are apolitical to the extent that they are neither associated with a particular political party nor do they call for wider political change such as more open, pluralist decision making, freedom of information or decentralisation.

A third conclusion would be that the relationship between the state, health professionals and other interested parties is crucial both in terms of the nature of any eventual policies (who is primarily responsible) and their likelihood of success. How these factors have combined historically will provide a large part of the explanation for the policies of the 1980's. This is the subject of the next three chapters.

4   1900–1945

Health professionals have argued that to combat heart disease in the 1980's the government should have a national policy which affects the diets of everyone (ie. the whole population) and which would change the national diet for health reasons alone. In other words they want the government to do as they suggest and to incur such disapproval as might emanate from, for example, farmers or food manufacturers. There have been examples in the past when elite professionals have been in a position to make similar suggestions and the object of this chapter is to see how successful these professionals have been in persuading the state to accept their suggestions in the past. Equally, it will be useful to know if these suggestions are more likely to be accepted under one set of conditions rather than another and what other factors (besides health) have been taken into consideration.

None of this represents an end in itself; it is only useful in the extent to which it can inform our understanding and explanation of policy decisions which have been taken in the past ten years or so. In these terms the justification for taking the approach I have outlined is simple. If elite professionals have never had any influence over the national diet from 1900-45 then this may affect our expectations of them doing so now.

Furthermore, if the state has never had such an interest, or was interested only at certain times, then this may account for the lack of professional influence more recently. On the other hand, if it is possible to discern an historical pattern of influence then this too would help any explanations if the pattern were to continue in the post World War Two period.

I want to argue in this chapter that there is such a pattern and that it can be found in five consistent features of policy making in the food and health field which have persisted throughout this period. Very briefly these are; 1. that the state will only intervene in the food supply of the whole population in times of actual, or expected, scarcity; 2. at other times the state will confine itself to supplementing the diets of the vulnerable sections of the population; 3. that there has always been administrative and political divisions of responsibility between food and health; 4. that the market status of food has figured prominently in any state intervention, whether in a crisis or not; and 5. that the price of food has always been central to its ability to supply the nutritional needs of the population. This list is by no means exhaustive but it does introduce the major themes of this, and the following chapter.

Historical comparisons are always going to be imperfect, however, there are certain features of the diet and heart disease controversy which suggest a starting point. To begin with, there is now a new body of knowledge which is of practical value and can be politically applied. Secondly, this knowledge has implications for the whole population and thirdly, there are very good reasons for applying this knowledge. This is very much the situation that existed during the First World War but, to fully appreciate this, I need to begin a little before 1914.

1900-1914

This sections looks at three examples of the British state taking an interest in the food supply of the population, or very large sections of it. I hope that it will become clear that, at this time, there were very particular circumstances under which the state was willing to do this. `ll of these examples refer to an expected or potential crisis for the state (i.e. war and a potential food scarcity). Equally, they highlight the market position of food, as opposed to its status as nutrients, and this in turn draws our attention to many of the structural constraints that were perceived to exist both by the state and by professionals. The first of these examples is the report of the *Interdepartmental Committee on Physical Deterioration* (1904).

During the Boer War (1900-1902), the director of the army medical services (Sir William Taylor) had expressed concern over the health of volunteers for the war. He had said that the Inspector of Recruiting was having difficulty in finding volunteers who were well enough to fight (Burnett;1979,p271). Approximately 40 per cent were rejected because of heart defects, bad hearing, eyesight and teeth. Even though the Royal College of Surgeons saw little point in pursuing the matter, an *Inter Departmental Committee on Physical Deterioration* was convened and reported in 1904. The fact that this committee was convened at all is interesting in itself. As Burnett said:

> The disclosures of poverty by Booth and Rowntree had
> little effect in government circles. More disturbing to
> Whitehall had been the admission ..that.. [there] .. was
> ....great difficulty in obtaining sufficient men of
> satisfactory physique for service in the forces;
> (Burnett;1979,p271).

> Because the government now had an interest in the
> physical condition of the population, the committee was
> duly appointed. There seems to have been a consensus
> on the root cause of the problem: "....all the witnesses
> concurred in giving the first place to food
> (Interdepartmental;1904,p59)".

The report established that there were a number of reasons for the malnourishment of volunteers. Ignorance, a decline in breast feeding and the abuse and adulteration of milk were all cited as reasons for the inadequate diets of many people. The Committee argued that the state did have a role to play in ameliorating the worst consequences of poverty, and recommended that the focus of attention should be schools:

> ...the period of school life offers the state its
> only opportunity for taking stock of the physique of
> the whole population and securing to its profit the
> conditions most favourable to healthy development
> (Interdepartmental;1904,p59).

The "profit" to the state was, presumably, the ability to raise an army when necessary and it is interesting to note that it was strategic considerations which were the motivation behind both the report and the subsequent policy initiatives. The Education (Provision of Meals) Act of 1906 was a direct result of this report and allowed local authorities to add one halfpenny in the pound (sterling) to the rates in order to provide school meals. By 1914 about 200,000 school children were receiving these meals as well as free dental and health care (Burnett;1979,p272).

It was no coincidence that the school was chosen as the best place for the state to intervene, or that children rather than adults were the focus of attention. Clearly the period of school life cannot be said to provide the "only" opportunity to secure a healthy population for there were many different ways of achieving this even in 1904. However, where welfare schemes did exist, whether state run or charitable, they were heavily orientated towards mothers, infants and children. For example, health visitors for pregnant women and nursing mothers, and school meals provided by the Friendly Societies. Given that these procedures already existed and needed only to be extended or institutionalised, the recommendations of the committee are understandable. In other words, the intention was to supplement and extend schemes which already existed, rather than create something which was entirely new. Of course, this does not detract from their intrinsic merit but it does give some indication not only of the parameters within which the solutions to such problems were discussed at this time but also of the reasons for the subject reaching the political agenda in the first place.

The Royal Commission on the Supply of Food and Raw Materials in Wartime (1905) is another example which supports many of the contentions and observations above. The report is interesting in a number of respects. One is that it was the strategic dimension or "potential crisis" which prompted the state into considering its role with regard to food, just as in the case above. Another, which is implicit in the Report on Physical Deterioration, is the relationship that was seen to exist between the state and the market. In the 1905 report there is a very strong feeling that if the market were protected from the commercial uncertainties of war then it could be relied upon to supply whatever the war effort might need. Consequently, it was not thought necessary to stockpile food but rather "...look mainly for security to the strength of our navy" (Royal Commission;1905) as this would protect imports. The Commission recommended that a National Indemnity scheme should be introduced to compensate traders who lost shipping because of the war. However:

...we do regard with concern the effect of war on

prices, and especially therefore on the conditions of the
poorer classes (Royal Commission;1905,p59).

The relationship between the price of food and the consumers ability to pay
for it was as obvious in 1905 as it is today. The Commission's worry was
that if food supplies could not be maintained, then not only would this
reduce the absolute amount of food for sale, but it would also raise the price
of the food that was available. Because imports accounted for
approximately two thirds of Britain's food, the emphasis on the
"strength of the navy" does not seem unreasonable. What may be
unreasonable is the fact that very little else was done. No specific
recommendations were made on the price of food in the main report;
there was, however, a minority report which criticised the complacency of
the report on food stocks, war prices, trade protection and other matters
(Royal Commission;1905,p65).

Here again, there are very particular circumstances under which the
state will consider its position with regard to the provision of food to
the whole population. When it did there is a very clear indication of the
legitimate boundaries of state action even in an expected crisis. The division
of responsibilities between the state and the market were very clearly
defined with the state simply trying to achieve the conditions in which the
free market could function efficiently. The only aspect of this market
which was thought to be problematical was the possibility of rising prices
and falling supplies and the remedy was seen as simply keeping the market
going. Clearly, however, this was a contentious area in 1905 and many of
the arguments are reminiscent of those heard today.

This relationship between supply and price can also be found in the last
example of this period. Beveridge, in his history of *British Food Control*
showed how unprepared Britain was for WW1 in terms of food supply and
control. He refers to the "War Book" (Beveridge;1928,p5) which laided
out contingency plans that were to be implemented by government
departments at the outbreak of war. With regard to food the book had only
one rule which was for Labour Exchanges to gather retail food prices,
which would in turn give an indication of regional food availability.
The assumption was that the level of supply in the various parts of the
country could be gauged by their food prices. As Starling said:

> For the most part, the provisioning of the nation has
> been regarded as an economic question to be solved by
> the laws of supply and demand (Starling;1919,p2).

As a scientist Starling was not only complaining about the lack of state intervention in food supply in the early years of WW1, but also about the lack of scientific input into policies. This is another theme that will be developed throughout this chapter but which is particularly evident during this period. The emerging body of scientific knowledge on dietary questions had not been related to the diets of large numbers of people. Even when planning for a war which threatened much of the country's food supplies, the state was not prepared to look beyond market forces to meet that supply. The state's role in the market would be transitory and minimalist in theory if not in practice during WWI and would, as far as possible, provide for the pre-war diet of the population. Initially this did not have any scientific basis but was based on pre-war production and consumption.

However, one state response to these scientific developments was the funding of the Medical Research Committee (later the Medical Research Council) in 1911, and its enquiry into the causes of rickets. It was later discovered that this disease was caused by a vitamin deficiency. Even so, as Drummond pointed out when referring to the 1904 report on Physical Deterioration :

> The doctors were completely obsessed with the quantitative outlook on dietary problems. Every problem was regarded in the light of the amount of protein or the total number of calories thought to be necessary (Drummond;1964,p231).

Perhaps it is fortunate, then, that at this stage (that is, without a thorough knowledge of vitamins and minerals) that such a 'marriage' had not taken place. And it is not surprising that it had not given the ideological disposition of the state to the market, the accepted peacetime role of the state with regard to food and the degree of welfare provision by the state as opposed to charities.

What is interesting about this period is not that the state did not immediately provide for the needs of the poor, adopt scientific evidence, intervene wherever nutritionally necessary in the market and co-opt scientists. It would have been unreasonable to have expected this. What is interesting are the circumstances under which the state *was* prepared to act, and how it envisaged acting. There was clearly some recognition of, and concern over, the diets of whole classes of the population. It was easier to accommodate school meals into the existing policies and the existing division of responsibilities; and they were easily assimilated into the general commitment to the vulnerable sections of society.

At the end of this section there are certain observations that can be made about the relationship between food, health and the state. During this period, the state was unwilling to extend its historical responsibility for maintaining the purity and integrity of food in response to the new nutritional knowledge. As Starling observed; "The provision of food for the nation was recognised to be the prime duty of government" only when there was a "threat of scarcity" (Starling;1919,p6). Similarly, the role of the market was seen as crucial to the continued supply of food even in a "crisis", the only anticipated problem with which might be the rise in food prices. At this stage then, the existence of such a threat (crisis) appears to be the only time that "population" approach to the supply of food was considered.

The First World War

In the previous section the examples I gave all dealt with the states' attempts to meet a potential or perceived crisis. This section looks at the actual crisis of the First World War. Many of the same themes are continued; in particular, the reluctance of the state to interfere in the market and the importance of the price of food to the level of overall supply. The existence of war does provide an opportunity to test the extent to which these factors constrained the states' actions or constituted part of the paradigm within which problems were considered. In addition, professionals were introduced into policy making and this was also important. I want to argue in this section that the role of the market in providing food was never seriously questioned in WWI, and it was only when the market appeared incapable of functioning properly, that the state intervened. I will further argue that exactly the same can be said of the state's use of professionals or experts. Their utility was that they could help solve the problems caused by a malfunctioning market; this implies that, in the absence of this malfunction, professionals would have been of considerably less use:

> The 1914-18 war provided the first occasion in history when the scientist was in a position to study such [nutritional] problems by precise methods and offer advice on their solution (Hollingsworth;1964,p431) .

70

Even so, having this ability was not in itself a sufficient reason for the state to ask for, or accept, that advice. Hollingsworth continued:

> The application of nutritional science to the problem of feeding the British population has been accelerated by national danger (1964,p431).

Hollingsworth's assumption is, of course, that WW1 merely acted as a catalyst to this application and that sooner or later it would have happened anyway. Obviously it is impossible to know one way or the other whether this is true or not, although the experiences of WW1 suggests that it might not be, given the evident reluctance of war-time governments to interfere in the operation of the market.

At the outbreak of war some government action was unavoidable. To begin with, Britain was in the unfortunate position of importing two thirds of its sugar from Austro-Hungary. The threat to supply that came with war caused panic buying and rapid price increases early in August 1914. This led to the government making large purchases of sugar later that month. By August 20th a Royal Commission on Sugar Supplies had been established which had the novelty of executive powers. Its terms of reference were:

> ...to inquire into the supply of sugar in the United Kingdom; to purchase, sell and control the delivery of sugar on behalf of the government, and generally take such steps as may be desirable for regulating the supply (Beveridge;1928,p6).

The apparent complacency of the Royal Commission into the Supply of Food and Raw Materials was not entirely unfounded in these early years of war. The Board of Trade (BoT), which was then responsible for food supply, did very little and the market continued to provide food in the way the Commission had expected.

Where intervention was necessary the profit margins of trade interests were assured. For example, when the government requisitioned "insulated" space on ships returning to Britain with meat supplies it would guarantee a certain price for the use of that space. Similarly, many of the new trading relationships which had to be established because of the war were kept secret from those involved. The government did not want any section of industry to acquire a competitive advantage that could be used after the war. It was not uncommon, therefore, for a producer not to know who the distributor of their goods was (Lloyd;1924,p325). Food prices did rise by some 25 percent in the first six months of war, but the remedy for this was deemed to be higher wages rather than any intervention in the market. On the whole then it was "business mainly as usual"; food was considered only one of many indices of inflation, and intervention in the structure and functioning of the market was kept to an absolute minimum. This was also the case with agricultural production which was essentially left to itself in the first two years of war.

By mid to late 1916 the situation was not quite the same and it began to take the form of a crisis that could not be resolved by the market. Food prices were now some 59 percent above their 1914 level, and although this may have been partly offset by there being little unemployment and larger numbers of women in the workforce, this did not allay criticisms in the press, parliament and the trade unions. As Coller put it:

> While the supply of food had to the present [June 1916] been adequate for the support of the population, the rises in prices had accentuated the inequalities of distribution, which reduced the daily ration to something below the level of efficiency (Coller;1925,p18).

Efficiency, measured as a persons ability to do work, was also a major theme of a report commissioned from the Royal Society's Physiological (War) Committee in June 1916 (Royal Society;1916). This committee constituted the expert advisory body for the government and was supplemented with an adviser who was attached to the cabinet. The committee, which eventually attached itself to the BoT, reported that while the supply of food was not substantially different from that before the war, distribution was becoming a problem. It also added its voice to the calls for greater controls over the food supply when it said:

> If the rising prices curtail for any class of the community its accustomed supply of food, its output of work will of necessity, be reduced (Royal Society;1916,p18).

The assumptions here are that 1. the accustomed supply was adequate, and 2. that it was the previous diet that should be replicated in the future. Neither of these assumptions were necessarily either correct or desirable in the light of the Interdepartmental report that was considered above. What this does indicate, however, is that the "experts" or elite professionals were not looking for radical solutions to the problems presented by the war; they were interested in copying the previous diets, not changing them radically. This became increasingly difficult as the war progressed, because the same food was simply not available.

It seems quite clear that at this stage the voice of those wanting a scientific approach to the supply of food was only one of many calling for greater intervention by the state. It is equally clear that until October and November of 1916 these calls were largely ignored. Beveridge has argued that this can be partly explained by the fact that Walter Runciman, the President of the BoT, was strongly anti-interventionist, and this is borne out by a speech he made in the House of Commons in October 1916:

> I have listened to the previous speakers......,all the time
> hungering and thirsting for business proposals
> (Runciman;1916).

While Runciman may well have been responsible for the timing of intervention, I would argue that the paradigm within which decisions were taken on food and the market was such that structural economic considerations were inevitable whoever was leading the BoT. This is primarily because the means of producing and distributing food were in private hands and because the British state had historically supported economic liberalism. Consequently, anyone in Runciman's position would have felt these constraints, but equally, would have found it necessary to intervene in the market at some stage.

The following month (November 1916) a food department was created within the BoT and by December there was a Ministry with a food controller. These events were the culmination of many things. In June, for example, the Interdepartmental Committee on Food Prices had worried about profiteering; there had been a bad potato crop; there were two parliamentary debates on food in October and November; and, of course, there were still highly vocal critics of the government both inside and outside of parliament.

Whatever the reasons for this shift in attitude, the beginning of 1917 and a new government headed by Lloyd George, saw the creation and integration of many political structures concerned with food. Figure 4.0

may help to conceptualise this.I have included the newly created Board of Health and Local Government (BoHLG) even though it did not, as far as I am aware, have any responsibilities for food except those associated with welfare. I have done this for a number of reasons. Firstly, from the outset the BoHLG (which was the predecessor of the Ministry of Health in 1919) was plagued with debates as to whether it should be integrated at national level and how its responsibilities should be divided up. This debate involved the Local Government Board, the Board of Education and the National Insurance Commission (Honigsbaum;1970). Interestingly, the medical profession were strongly against the formation of a Ministry of Health or any centralised form of executive control over their work. This is reminiscent of the approach they adopted to the formation of the National Health Service.

Fig.4.0.

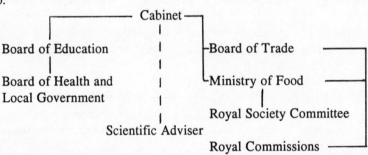

The important things to recognise at this stage are that the administering of health policies necessarily requires some decentralisation and local administration whether it be for hospitals, health visitors or clinics. Before the arrival of the NHS, charities and local authorities which operated at local level were largely responsible for this sort of thing, because service delivery must be localised. This is not necessarily the case for food policies. They are political constructs, and while in wartime they do require a vast machinery because they deal with all aspects of food, this need not be the case in peace. Secondly, the dichotomy that now exists between those responsible for diet/health and those responsible for food policies, is nothing new. There have always been separate structures for pricing, supply, distribution and production on the one hand, and for the health implications of those policies on the other.

There is no need to catalogue each act of food control but as Lloyd argues:

> The tendency.....was for more responsibility to be
> devolved to the traders themselves as control was
> gradually extended and as the idea of cooperation
> between private trade and the government began to
> replace the necessity of compulsion (1924,p363).

Again, the voluntarist principle is at the core of many of these arrangements. Trades were not, in general, particularly well organised before the war and the need for cooperation both between traders and between traders and the state, accelerated a tendency that had been evident but not substantial, before the war.

The principle, then, was to try ,as far as possible, not to interfere in the market and, in particular, not to give any advantages to individual traders, although the more efficient traders inevitably did better.

The advent of stricter food controls changed the relationship between the state and the consumer as well. The need for consumers to trust the MoF was interpreted by the officials as meaning a more "above the board" approach to decision making so that the actions and motives of the Ministry would not be misunderstood or misinterpreted by consumers. It was this laudable principle which was responsible for the Ministry publishing a food journal and establishing the Food Consumers Council (Dec 1917).[1] It is interesting to see that as the state extended its responsibilities with regard to food many other familiar aspects of policy making began to emerge as a consequence. Consumer representation, voluntarism and the incorporation of experts are all things which exist today because the state has accepted a particular degree of involvement in the supply of food.

I think it is reasonable to say that the first 6 months of 1917 brought with it fairly haphazard attempts at food control, involving the voluntary rationing of meat and bread and meatless days in restaurants. Beveridge argues that it was only when Rhondda was appointed to the Ministry of Food, that science was incorporated into policies. Rhondda certainly appears to have been predisposed to incorporating professional opinion into policy, but the circumstances in which he found himself as food controller were probably equally as important in determining his use of this advice.

The notion that science was a basis for policies became a publicity point when voluntary ration levels were set in September 1917. The MoF

---

[1] The representation on the council was: 6 members of the cooperative movement; 9 TUC; and 3 taxpayers (Beveridge;1928,p71).

emphasised that the levels, which were consistent with the League of National Safety guidelines, were "highly scientific". Nevertheless, changing personal and commercial habits simply because they were contrary to scientific advice was as big a problem then as it is now. For instance, farmers were extremely reluctant to slaughter their cattle earlier than usual simply because experts thought this would reduce herds and feedstuffs.

Politically those who advised on the nutritional aspects of food supply were in a weak position. While Beveridge was able to say that their advice was never ignored, it is also true to say that there was little opportunity for any permanent physical presence in decision making and there was certainly no form of sanction available to experts who were ignored. In WWI, as in WWII, science was listened to and accommodated where expedient and practicable. At the end of World War One the Ministry of Food was dismantled and there was a general desire to return to normality.

To conclude this section I want to draw out some of the more obvious points. The first of these is that both before and during the War, the state's attitude toward food consumption and the nature of the food supply was coloured by food's commodity status and by its nutritional value. Having this commodity status meant that the place of food in the market, and the many commercial relationships which put it there, were protected and encouraged. The value of the food in nutritional terms was only important if the market failed to operate normally. These then are the circumstances under which the state will affect the food supply of the whole population. Before the war, welfare was targetted at those sections of the population for whom there was an effective scarcity because either income or price restricted supply. Finally, the First World War saw professionals incorporated into the decision making process on a temporary basis. Professionals were used as problem solvers, and as such, were useful only as long as the state perceived those problems to exist.

The Inter-War Years

The scale of state intervention in the economy that had been necessary during WWI was unprecedented and, on the whole, the state was willing to retreat to its pre-war position of non-intervention. However, the depression of the late 1920's and early 1930's renewed pressure on the state to abandon free-trade and to protect British industry. This depression affected food supplies to the extent that it produced abject poverty and it raised the price of food. The inter-war years, therefore, provide an example of a "perceived or articulated crisis" for the state (economic depression) but without the state taking the degree of responsibility for the food supply which occurred in the First World War. It is also an interesting time because the bearers of the "new" knowledge on nutrition became much more vociferous in their condemnation of governments and in their belief that their science should be incorporated into public policy. Consequently, there is an intensification of many of the themes and ideas introduced so far, and an opportunity to consider them under peace-time conditions.

The tendency for trades to associate continued between the wars and led to the number of trade associations rising from 500 in 1919 to approximately 2,500 in 1939 (see: Skuse;1976,p150 also, Aldcroft;1983 and Pollard;1983). Retailing and distribution expanded even through the depression and there were the beginnings of the "multiples" which were gradually replacing the specialist shops. Many of the larger food firms such as Ranks, Liptons and Spillers which had benefited from the war, also expanded. The industry was healthy in the interwar years largely because of the nature of its products; the income elasticity of demand for food is quite low (particularly for staple products such as bread) and in consequence the industry did not suffer to the extent that other manufacturing and retail sectors did.

But it was the rise of nutrition as a science capable of solving health and social problems which changed the character of the debate between professionals and the state. The inter-war years were the golden age of nutrition. During this time most of the major vitamins and minerals were identified and, equally importantly, their effects were studied. Much of this research was carried out under the auspices of the Medical Research Council, a government funded body. There were many aspects to this work ranging from the production of synthetic vitamins to determining what the effects of vitamin deficiencies might be (Landsborough;1975,p80). This new knowledge provided professionals with a sound basis upon which to assess the health of the population in nutritional terms. It is a relatively small step from knowing what is good about a food or nutrient, to criticising what is bad and many of these criticisms are similar to those heard today. Boyd-Orr, the first director of the United Nations Food and Agriculture Organisation (FAO), was an outspoken critic of British food. In 1933 he spoke of foods "no longer being natural" and gave the examples of "polished rice, white flour, sugar, dried milk and tinned foodstuffs." He went on to say:

The natural foods have been changed into artificial foods with the very substances purified away that were necessary to perfect health (Lancet;1933,p657).

It was also Boyd-Orr who wrote one of the most influential and contentious studies of the nutritional status of the British population; *Food, Health and Income* (Boyd-Orr;1936). This study looked at the adequacy of the diets of a sample of the population and correlated this with their incomes. It was Boyd-Orr's contention that many people in Britain in the 1930's simply did not have the income to purchase an adequate diet. By dividing the sample into income groups, he found the following:

Group 1. (4.5 million people). Diets were inadequate in all areas.
Group 2. (9.0 million people). Diets were adequate only in total proteins and fats.
Group 3. (9.0 million people). Diets adequate in total energy (calories), protein and fats.
Group 4. (9.0 million people). Diets are adequate but a probable calcium deficiency.
Group 5. (9.0 million people). Only the possibility of a calcium deficiency.
Group 6. (4.5 million people). No deficiencies (Boyd-Orr;1936,p36-37).

There are a number of points that should be made about this. The most obvious is that this type of study, which attempts to quantify the dietary inadequacies within a population, is only possible when inadequacies can be quantified, that is, when professionals know what an adequate diet might be. To this extent, then, Boyd-Orr's study relied upon the existence of that knowledge. Secondly, by establishing the relationship between "Food, Health and Income" Boyd-Orr was arguing that there were causes of ill health which were, in essence, structural to the consumer; ie. income. As a consequence of this, even though it may be possible to improve a persons diet by helping them to make better informed decisions, the solution to the problem must ultimately be political. Indeed, the political nature of the policy area was demonstrated when the Ministry of Health, which had supported Boyd-Orr's study, distanced itself from its findings.

When The Lancet (1936,p679-680) reviewed *Food, Health and Income* it repeated a telling observation that had been made by Boyd-Orr himself when it suggested that more than one government department would be responsible for the solution to these problems. This was, indeed, the case because questions of food production, protection and subsidy were primarily the responsibility of the Exchequer, the Board of Agriculture and Fisheries and the Board of Trade. Once again, the health consequences of the actions (or otherwise) of these departments remained with the Ministry of Health. There was no Ministry of Food which could act as an umbrella for any policy initiatives, nor, as was the case in Norway, a Food Council which could coordinate inter-departmental policies.

A National Food Council was one of the demands of the Committee Against Malnutrition which was formed in 1934. This committee, which counted Harold Macmillan amongst its number, wanted to see a council which had representatives of food producers and consumers as well as scientists. The objectives of the Council would be to formulate a national food policy. The committee was also critical of those policies which were designed to solve the problems of British agriculture by restricting the food supply (thus raising price) rather than expanding demand.

The problems faced by British agriculture between the wars revolved around the world over-capacity in food production and the fall in demand because of the depression. British agriculture found it impossible to compete with imports and in order to protect British farmers, import restrictions were imposed after the abandonment of free-trade in 1931 (Murray;1955,p26-29). This, of course, raised the price of food in Britain when, with a world glut, food prices should have been much lower. The policy seems, in retrospect at least, even more perverse because of the levels of unemployment and the obvious poverty that existed at the time. This was the basis of the criticism that came from the Committee Against Malnutrition; it would have been much more sensible to expand consumer demand and, by doing so, improve the national diet and the circumstances of British agriculture at the same time.

Despite the obvious need for nutritional and agricultural considerations to be taken together, there are very few examples of this happening during the inter-war period; in fact milk is the only example. There was a Standing Advisory Committee on Milk Production which serviced both the Ministry of Health and the Board of Agriculture, and which was set up following a recommendation by the 1923 Departmental Committee on Agricultural Prices (Spann;1940,p246). Milk had been recognised as a valuable food even during the First World War and the state had conceded to a National Milk Publicity Council which was followed by the Milk Marketing Board in 1933. Milk production suffered from the same problems as the rest of agriculture and in 1934 demand was 20% below the available supply. However, in 1934 the government provided £500,000 to publicise and subsidise milk (Elliot;1934,col 503-504). This followed a statement in the House of Commons by the Minister of Agriculture who said:

> An expansion of liquid milk consumption would not only be of the greatest benefit from the public health point of view but would alleviate in the most satisfactory way the difficulty of "surplus milk" (Elliot;1934,col 503-504).

The reluctance to intervene in the market on health grounds alone was shelved here primarily because of the coincidence of interests between milk producers and consumers.

It would be wrong to suggest that the state had no interest in nutrition or the expanding body of knowledge that was accumulating during this period. It is clear that this was not the case, but the application of this knowledge to the health of large sections of the population was another matter. In 1931 the Ministry of Health established the Advisory Committee on Nutrition which is the ancestor of the present Committee on the Medical Aspects of Food Policy (COMA). The terms of reference of this committee were:

> ...to inquire into the facts, quantitative and qualitative in relation to the diet of the people, and report as to any changes therein which appear desirable in the light of modern advances in the knowledge of nutrition (Hollingsworth;1985,p255).

This committee is the first example of professionals with nutritional knowledge being incorporated into the Ministry in an advisory capacity. While in principle the establishment of this committee was laudable, in practice, the committee provided the government with the means to counter many of the criticisms which the Ministry and the government were receiving. For example, in 1933 the British Medical Association published a report which argued that the average male required 3,400 calories a day. The Ministry and the League of Nations had both set the level at 3,000 calories a day and it was the Advisory committee which attended a special conference organised to settle the matter with the BMA in May 1934. The importance of the subject rested not only on the fact that the Ministry may have made a mistake, but also on the implications for assessing the health of the population. The discrepancies were methodological; the Ministry based its figure on whole communities and the BMA were primarily concerned

80

with the unemployed (Lancet;1934,p1098-1099).

The advisory committee did not report until 1937 and the report itself contrasted significantly with Boyd-Orr's study (which had been published the previous year) by arguing that the national diet was generally adequate although there was some room for improvement. It is difficult to escape the conclusion that, while the government had a legitimate interest in taking advice from an "official" source, this source played a political as well as a scientific role. This, in combination with the fact that there was very little interest in expanding government responsibilities on food beyond the welfare provision of milk in schools for example, suggests that at this stage nutrition was a secondary consideration in food-related policies.

Despite the opportunities that were available to the state to manipulate import restrictions and subsidies on health grounds, these opportunities were not taken. By and large, questions of food remained commercial questions rather than health questions. The exception, as might be expected, is found in the vulnerable sections of the population. It was they that benefited from the welfare supplies of milk. Again, it can be argued that the 1920's and the 1930's represented a crisis for the British state and it is for this reason alone that any intervention in the food supply was considered. Similarly, the response of the state was to enlist and incorporate professionals and experts into the decision making process as it had done in 1916. The difference during the inter-war years appears to be that the role of these professionals was as much political as it was practical.

The Second World War

The final section of this chapter looks at the Second World War. The format of this section is roughly the same as in the others; we are looking to see what the determinants of population level strategies on nutrition have been and how influential professionals are in determining, on health grounds, the nature of the food supply. The Second World War is the most serious example of expected food scarcity that the modern British state has faced. Under these circumstances, it would not be unreasonable to expect that professionals were elevated to a much more prominent role with regard to the food supply. In comparison to the other periods this is, indeed, the case. Nevertheless, the main themes that have been visible throughout this chapter still hold true. I want to argue in this section that "science" and/or professionals were only one of many policy inputs and that, while they enjoyed some influence over the details of policy, they were largely excluded from attempts to plan the food supply during the Second World War.

The system of welfare provision of foods was actually extended during the war. Priority supplies of milk were available to the under fives and expectant mothers; there was an expansion of the milk in schools scheme which had begun before the war; the school meals scheme was also expanded; children aged between six months and two years were given priority rations of eggs; and cod liver oil and concentrated orange juice were available, again for children and expectant mothers (Hollingsworth;1985,p255). While it may seem surprising, on one interpretation at least, that during a war the amount of expenditure on welfare should increase on another level it should be less surprising. As I have said above, the state has been predisposed to cater for these vulnerable sections of the population during times of crisis. While the extent and nature of these provisions may indicate a degree of elite or professional influence over public policy, a far better test from our point of view, is the extent to which scientists, nutritionists or health professionals were able to influence the food supply to the whole population during the war. This would give a much better indication of the circumstances under which such opinions would be incorporated into policy and, by inference, the likelihood of incorporation.

Prior to the Second World War (1936) the Food (Defence Plans) Department of the Board of Trade had studied the question of wartime food supplies (Hammond;1951,p218). The board had organised contingency plans for the war and received assurances from trade interests that they would cooperate, particularly in building up food stocks (Hammond;1951,p20). However, Beveridge, who had worked in the Ministry of Food in the First War, was unable to convince the committee that they should detail exactly which foods should be grown in wartime and in what quantities. With this failure vanished any chance of experts planning wartime food supplies. As Hammond observed in his official history:

> It is emphatically not the case.. that food policy was
> scientifically determined from the outbreak of the war,
> or indeed at any time (Hammond;1951,p44).

Leaving aside for the moment the difficulties surrounding what constitutes "determining" a policy given the uncertainties of war, a strong case can, nevertheless, be made to support the argument that despite the experiences of the first world war and the large body of scientific

82

knowledge of nutrition then available, it took some time for scientists to be installed in the decision making processes concerned with food.

Indeed, in April 1940 Dr Edith Summerskill was moved to ask in the House of Commons:

> Why had not the problem of food supply been approached in an entirely different way, and why had not someone with a knowledge of food values been consulted? (Lancet;1940,p713).

At this time butter, bacon, ham, sugar, and meat were already rationed and food subsidies of one million pounds (sterling) per week were set on bread, flour, meat, milk, and bacon. There was a "Chief Scientific Adviser" to the Ministry of Food (Jack Drummond) who was appointed in February 1940 and who had previously been adviser on food contamination, but the various sections within the Ministry had developed around certain types of foods (these were, and are, called commodity divisions) and were operating on an ad hoc basis.

In June 1940 a Scientific Food Committee (SFC) was appointed in response to a report from the Select Committee on Public Expenditure which criticised the piecemeal development of the commodities divisions within the MoF. The Public Expenditure Committee recommended that the SFC's job should be to work out a basic plan for wartime food policy. There was also some concern over the possibility that the commodity divisions might be protecting the interests of the trades they represented (Lancet;1940,p971).

By the end of 1941 the SFC had been replaced by the Ministry of Health's Inter-Departmental Committee on Medical and Nutritional Problems. The MoF still retained a scientific resource because a Scientific Advisers Division had joined the commodities division within the Ministry itself in 1942.

Even so, this was not seen as sufficient by many people. In late 1942 The Lancet (1942,p399-401), in a leading article, was calling for a Nutrition Council to coordinate the efforts of the Ministries of Food, Health, Agriculture and Education.

The scientists within the Ministry of Food appear to have seen the war as providing an opportunity for changing the diet of the nation permanently. However, they were confronted with the wartime expediency of the departmental officials. The "basal diet" had been formulated at the beginning of the war to provide a minimum subsistence diet to the British people. It relied heavily upon the use of cereals and vegetables and, as such, would have transformed not only the British diet, but also the pattern of British agriculture. Officials within the Ministry of Food wanted to see this diet "put to sleep for the duration of the war". As Hammond observed:

> The scientists were indignant; they felt that the officials had usurped their function in pronouncing on the ends as well as the means of food policy. They protested against the implication that "consumption....should be adjusted to the results of the existing system of guarantees and subsidies rather than the latter adjusted to ensure the quantities which scientific research shows to be desirable", and they read into the arguments of the officials a wish to superimpose the food production campaign on the pre-war pattern of British Agriculture; rather than change that pattern radically (Hammond;1951,p95).

The system of guarantees had been agreed between the government and the farmers within the first months of the war and, as I mentioned earlier, the subsidies had been set in early 1940. Furthermore, the Scientific Food Committee suffered from a remoteness from the day to day experiences of the Departments where policy was being made, it was thus difficult for it to gain an overall perspective on policy or to exercise the influence that it might have wished (Hammond;1951,p96).

It seems, then, that there was some disparity between what the "experts" wanted to achieve and what the officials thought their role should be. It is difficult to establish not only whether this disparity actually had an effect on wartime food policies, but equally, what the overall vision of the scientists was at this time. Boyd-Orr however was quite clear when he wrote:

> That problem [of malnutrition] will never be solved until our national food policy is based on the food requirements of the people and not on the interests of trade as it has been in the past (Boyd-Orr;1940,p6).

He went on to complain about the vigorous rationing of protective foods and fixing prices at a level too high for the poor to afford. The inference appears to be that vested interests (from either the state, agriculture or the "trades") should be compelled to perform in accordance with scientifically prescribed goals. These goals would re-structure production and pricing on the basis of what Britain could produce itself and what the population needed to remain nutritionally well-provided for.

Certainly it would seem that in the early years of the war at least, science and scientists were "structurally disadvantaged" in relation to agricultural and food industry interests. The Minister of Agriculture was a former President of the National Union of Farmers and the head controllers of the commodities divisions of the Ministry of Food for butter, cereals, feedingstuffs, tea, canned fish, meat and livestock, bacon and ham, dried fruits, sugar, imported eggs, potatoes, oils and fats and condensed milk were all taken from those particular industries or ones similar in nature (Darling;1941,p59). All these appointments combined the administrative virtue of continuity between the state and those it relied upon to implement such things as pricing and distribution policies, with the disadvantage of fostering a conflict of interests for those appointed. This conflict was recognised as being potentially damaging both to the war effort and to the health of the general public. The most cited example of this concerned increasing the amount of flour that was produced from wheat (Lancet;1942,p337).

In agriculture both a quantitative and a qualitative approach was necessary in the production of food. The Ploughing Up Campaign, which began very early in the war, was clearly necessary to the extent that imports could be expected to fall. Equally, however, *what* was grown was also important, because the extra production would need to nutritionally replace the imports that were being lost. The experience of WW1 was useful in that there was a determination to reduce the size of cattle herds in favour of arable farming, and priority was given to dairy herds.

Even so there was some controversy as to the extent to which the herds should be reduced given the uncertainties surrounding the feedingstuffs available. The argument revolved around the need to maintain milk output which the Scientific Food Committee and the Economics Division of the Ministry of Food believed required slaughtering large numbers of cattle to save grass and feed and to release meat. The Ministry of Agriculture and the Meat and Livestock Division of the MoF were against this policy saying that it was unnecessary and possibly harmful to farmers. Those incentives that were introduced to encourage early slaughter do not appear to have overridden the reluctance of farmers to slaughter good animals. In addition, the maintenance of cattle herds did not appear to affect the overall output of milk in the way that had been expected (ie. to reduce it) so the farmers conservatism was not entirely unfounded (Hammond;1951,p176). Regardless of the merits, or otherwise, of these arguments   this is a good example of the difficulties faced in manipulating agricultural production and in having this division of responsibility for food scattered   between so many interested parties. This may partially explain why agricultural expansion at the beginning of the war was based largely on "the pre-war pattern". The relationship that existed between food and agriculture is succinctly expressed by Hammond:

> ...the Minister of Food might state his requirements
> from home production,..... The Ministers responsible
> for agriculture must say how far and in what way those
> requirements might be supplied (Hammond;1951,p179).

This appears to confirm both that production was not "scientifically determined" from the outset and that the Ministry of Food was not in the position to demand of the Ministry of Agriculture "heroic" changes in the pattern of production.

Nevertheless, the ploughing up campaign doubled the acreage under wheat and potatoes by the end of the war. There was a 45% increase in vegetable output, a doubling of oats and barley and a halving of food imports (Burnett;1979,p323).   It would be wrong, and unnecessary, to suppose that all these decisions were made without reference to any person, or group of people who could be classed as professionals. The increase in carrot and potato acreage was achieved on "expert" advice. Equally, many of the foods chosen for import under the lend lease scheme were chosen on nutritional grounds; the most obvious example being dried eggs. My argument is simply that there was always a political and bureaucratic context in which these decisions were made and that professionals could never be seen as being dominant, even in wartime.

Agricultural prices were set by the Ministry of Agriculture while the price of food was the responsibility of the MoF within the broad policy of pegging the cost of living index at something approaching 30% above its 1939 level.   This was something agreed to by the Inter Departmental Committee on Food Prices in 1940. Again, as in WWI, food prices were determined not only by their nutritional value, but by their position in the economy as a whole.

Figure 4.1 is an attempt to clarify the inputs into food policy during

WW11 after they had settled down in late 1942.

Fig 4.1.

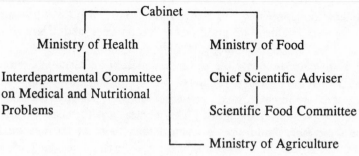

By this time there was a regular pattern of consultation on imports between the scientists and the officials and a checks and balances system for the approval of decisions concerning food which involved three separate committees, often reaching cabinet level. It is clearly the case that food required a great deal of coordination between various departments before policies were put into action. Equally, at various places in these separate but inter-related structures interests were harmonised by the desire on the part of the state to provide sufficient food at prices that were affordable. Indeed, ultimately all interests were harmonised by the desire to win the war. In this respect, the position of the state, and its relationship with these various interests took on a character that was unique to war time.

Given the complexity of the task in hand, the conflicting interests that were involved in the policy process and the constraints of the war economy, it was a major achievement to have secured food which, in calorific terms at least, approached pre-war levels. There were also many legacies of WWII; the Food Standards Committee; the eventual amalgamation of the Ministries of Agriculture and Food; the extended welfare provisions to mothers and children were retained; a consolidated policy on agriculture; and a scientific division within MAFF. All of these differentiate WWII from WWI.

Professionals certainly had a role to play but there were other compelling factors which diluted their influence. One was that they were late-comers to the plans that were made at the beginning of the war; another was the conservatism of farmers; yet another their remoteness from the practicalities of the decisions they were taking. War demands expediency and often the line of least resistance holds as much, if not more, compulsion to the administrator and policy maker as the most beneficial policy. Because of this, WWII both facilitated the application of science to policies concerning diet and health by providing occasions for inputs which had not previously existed; and it constrained them because food and diets were subject to multi-factoral influences and interests whose concerns had to be accommodated.

It is also interesting that there was a noticeable distinction between the "scientist" and the official particularly at the beginning of the war, each side viewing the problems (and their solutions) in different lights and according to varying paradigms. This contrasts with today's technocrats who are far more "ministry" orientated than those of the Second World War. It seems that there was little room for "grand designs" after 1942 and to that extent at least it would appear as though the pattern, as opposed to the details, of food control in WWII were set administratively rather than scientifically.

Conclusion

In the periods that I have looked at in this chapter I think that it is fairly clear that there are certain themes and consistencies in the states' response to the threats to the British food supply it has experienced.

One of these responses is that the state is generally unwilling or reluctant to intervene in the provision of food except where the operation of the market cannot be relied upon to provide for the nutritional needs of the people. It is interesting that the state has been far more willing to legislate in areas which promote free and fair trade in food, than in directing its production or consumption. This underlines the necessity of creating the right commercial conditions for the market to operate and, of course, a faith in the market to respond. Similarly, state aided welfare provision has existed in a modern form (ie post Poor Law) for most of this century simply because the market is demonstrably incapable of guaranteeing nutritional adequacy (amongst other things) for all. These represent a "bottom line" or "safety net" which is only exceeded by the state when the market itself comes under pressure and when its ability to provide either food or employment is threatened. Thus, the two world wars and the depression of the 1930's provoked a crisis which demanded state intervention in, or concern over, food supplies.

It is at these points of crisis that science appears more likely to be a major policy input. However,the nature of that input has tended to be transitory (ie. its eminence is confined to the crisis itself) and confined to problem solving rather than to planning long term solutions to persistent problems. To this extent, the prominence that science has enjoyed in influencing the nature of the British food supply has suffered in the long run because of the circumstances under which it was thought necessary to apply it. These circumstances have always been extraordinary and this has put professionals in a politically weak position in times of peace or non-crisis. The pattern of issues and policies which the state has left to professionals has therefore become highly predictable. As a consequence, crucial health considerations such as pricing, agricultural production, subsidies, import quotas and the like have been largely excluded from professional influence. This exclusion is reflected in the persistent departmental division of responsibilities between food, agriculture and health which has further undermined the political influence of professionals.

Again, when there has not been a crisis the responsibilities of the state have remained fairly consistent towards certain sections of the population. It is primarily expectant and nursing mothers, infants and school children who benefit directly from state intervention and provision in peacetime. The most vulnerable sections of society are protected because these are the sections which the market cannot accommodate ie. those that are unproductive. This protection has not been to the detriment of the market; the milk subsidies of the 1930's suggest that even welfare provision will be compatible with the needs of industry as well as the vulnerable.

Even so, those who are not "officially" vulnerable when there is not a crisis may not be as secure as public policy would have us believe. If food is a marketed commodity like any other, and if this status is assumed to be sufficient to provide for most peoples nutritional needs, then there are a number of other assumptions that follow from this. One is that what the food market actually provides is nutritionally adequate and that the price is affordable. A further assumption is that consumers know which foods are desirable and purchase accordingly.

Neither of these assumptions are necessarily correct and the major misfortune of this, as Boyd-Orr demonstrated, is that it is those who are not well informed or well off who are most likely to suffer whether there is a crisis or not. There are two other factors which aggravate this situation still further. The first is another assumption taken from the commodity status of food; ie. that leaving food supply almost entirely to the discretion of the market means that we must further accept that food producers, manufacturers and retailers will produce only those foods which can be sold. This does not necessarily mean that these foods are particularly valuable, only profitable. The second aggravating factor for the badly informed or badly-off is that there are times when received wisdom on what is good or bad food changes radically. At these times (the 1980's for example) even if consumers are trying to buy wisely, they may simply get it wrong. I would argue, on the basis of the above, that if, as has been the case in this chapter, food supply is left to the discretion of the market, then much greater control over price, information, education and availability would be required to achieve any given nutritional ends. It has only been in times of crisis that the state has remotely approached such a position.

The difficulties that are faced by those in contemporary Britain who demand "a" food policy or state intervention in the supply of food are now more clearly understood given historical precedent.

Explanations of particular policy outcomes in the past ten years or so obviously require more than this. It is clear from this chapter, however, that (1) anything approaching an integrated policy involving all sections of the food chain; (2) which requires actions by the state that is contrary to established interests within MAFF; (3) that furthermore uses science as its primary justification; and (4) does not build entirely or at least substantially on the existing policies, will have to overcome a great many structural, ideological and economic obstacles. The extent to which the themes and patterns of this chapter hold true or develop in the post-war period, is the subject of the following three chapters.

5 Food and Agriculture Since WWII

The politics of dietary change lies at the intersection of two, historically distinct, policy areas; food and health.   This intersection has become known as "nutrition" but there has been surprisingly little policy that can be called nutritional.   Most has been aimed at the vulnerable, (children, infants, mothers, the elderly etc), and not at the population as a whole.

The intersection is therefore important, because it denotes a point at which two policy areas meet with a mutual interest.   This chapter is primarily concerned with establishing what the interests on the "food" side are and how they have fitted in with post-war conceptions of nutrition.   The following chapter will look at health.   If we are going to explain policies on dietary change then it is clearly important to know about food and health and the interests that operate in these areas.   In this chapter we will consider the role of MAFF, the farmers and the food industry since WWII and discuss how they interact, and what they want from public policy.

Sectors and Sub-Sectors in Food and Agriculture

During the Second World War Britain had a food and nutrition policy which integrated questions of health, production and distribution. Although it was never "scientifically determined" it was nevertheless the closest Britain has come to a deliberate nutrition policy. The fate of that policy confirms one of the central contentions of the previous section, namely, that it is only when there is a threat or perceived threat to the aggregate level of food supply that the state will intervene in supply on health grounds. When the need for rationing was no longer with us, nor was an autonomous Ministry of Food.

To fully understand the pattern of relationships and the distribution of resources within MAFF we must consider food and agriculture at both the sectoral and the sub-sectoral level. This is more difficult than it appears because it is often difficult to distinguish between agricultural and food sectors, and because these relationships are extremely complex. Similarly, it is very difficult to talk of "a" sector which constitutes food processing in general, because it is a very diverse industry. Nevertheless, with care it is possible to make viable distinctions and to recognise those areas of policy which unify and divide food manufacturing, food retailing and agriculture.

The problems that were associated with food before the War were broadly of two types. The first were the age-old problems of fraud and safety, and had been accepted as the responsibility of the state since the 1860 Food and Drug Act. The second type of problem revolved around malnourishment caused primarily by insufficient incomes. As Boyd-Orr recognised, low incomes meant that many people were not receiving the vitamins and minerals which research between the wars had established were necessary for health. The experiences of the Second World War demonstrated that if income were controlled for, then the general level of health in the population could be maintained, if not improved (Hollingsworth;1985). Therefore, the scientific orthodoxy of the time argued that consumers should eat a varied and balanced diet and would then get all the essential nutrients they need.

It is not difficult to imagine that in the post-war period the problems of nutrition in western industrialised countries were widely thought to be solved. The science of nutrition turned its attention to the deficiency diseases of the third world and the perceived protein gap:

For most students in Oxford in those days [1947] there

were no remaining unsolved problems in human nutrition. All the necessary food factors had been identified. All that was necessary was to eat a good mixed diet, preferably three square meals daily, avoid obesity and all would be well. (Acheson;1986,p137).

Immediately after the war this advice was largely immaterial not only because Britain was still threatened with food shortages, but also because of its precarious finances. The ending of lend-lease and the dollar shortage not only curtailed Britain's ability to import food, it also ensured the continuation of policies designed to increase self sufficiency for the sake of the balance of payments and ultimately for the value of sterling.

Because these shortages still existed, so did the machinery of state intervention in the food supply:

> On Nov 7 1945, the Minister of Food announced that the Ministry of Food would be retained....ensuring that adequate supplies of food necessary for health were available to all members of the public at reasonable prices (Winnifrith;1962,p36).

The relationship between scarcity, health and state intervention was once again confirmed, as was the relationship between health and income (prices). However, as Robbins and Bowman have argued, WWII:

> ...was..a time when nutrition and food production were most closely related at the policy level: a relationship which was not maintained after the war (Robbins and Bowman;1983,p184).

Notwithstanding the continued commitment of the state to the safety of food which must, by definition, have a health component, Robbins and Bowmans' contention is an accurate description of how things emerged after the de-control of food in 1954. The transition from the integrated policy of the War, to this "divorce" is extremely important to any understanding of the rationale of post-war food policies and their compatibility with current recommendations on dietary change.

It has been well established that the basis of post-war food and agriculture policies were primarily strategic and economic in nature:

93

There was anxiety particularly about the balance of payments, and international food continued to be in short supply and expensive (Howarth;1985,p11).

It was accepted that the aim of agricultural policy must be to expand agriculture to its limits and that government had a role in ensuring that the incentives existed for farmers to carry out such a policy.....The policy of agricultural support and production was not questioned by any post-war government (Smith;1988,p14).

So, Britain needed to continue its wartime policy of maximising production and it did this by using the price guarantee system that had operated during the war. This was changed in 1953 to a system of deficiency payments which worked, largely unchanged, until Britain entered the EEC in 1973.

Table 5.0. Changes in output of given products 1945-1980.

Year	Milk million gallons	Eggs million dozen	Poultry million tons	Beef million tons	Sheep million tons	Pork million tons
1945	1.75	448	-	0.526	0.132	0.03
1955	2.25	800	0.18	0.66	0.18	0.46
1960	2.62	1043	0.30	0.73	0.23	0.79
1965	2.44	1215	0.41	0.88	0.26	0.92
1975	2.93	1117	0.65	1.21	0.27	0.82
1980	3.38	1100	0.76	1.19	0.28	0.95

Source: Holderness;1985,p174.

This meant that farmers were encouraged to produce as much as possible and, in particular, to produce those foods which could be grown in Britain. Table 5.0 testifies that this policy has been successful. The position of the National Farmers Union was also institutionalised in the 1947 Agriculture Act which assured them the right of consultation with the Ministry before prices were set (Wilson;1977,p42-3).

Until 1955, there was still a separate Ministry of Food which in some ways acted as a counter-weight to the Ministry of Agriculture, being, as it was, more consumer orientated. Consequently, there was a degree of inter-departmental pluralism. This distinction still exists today in that the Food Standards Division within MAFF tends to be the most consumer orientated of the divisions within MAFF.

The strength of the relationship between the Ministry of Agriculture and the farmers came about through the Annual Price Review which was the forum for setting the guaranteed prices (later the level of deficiency payment, and later still the intervention prices Britain would argue for in the EEC):

> The full import of this arrangement only emerged slowly. One effect was to place the government under strong pressure to attune its programme of support to the wishes of the union...[although the government reserved the right to make the final decisions]....a convention soon emerged whereby the union gave a formal endorsement of some kind to the final settlement (Self and Storing;1962,p63).

It seems clear, therefore, that production policies were geared to the maximisation of output and, as a consequence, entailed close political relationships between MAFF and the farmers which persist to this day.

During the War, the relationships between the various groups amounted to inter-departmental pluralism which meant that there was a tendency for interests to counter-balance one another. The establishment of the Annual Price review institutionalised the "exclusion" of consumer groups from agricultural pricing (Smith;1988) as it was a forum only for the Ministry and the NFU; even the Milk Marketing Board was excluded from the pricing of milk at that time. When rationing ended the balance of forces between the Ministries changed because the Ministries of Agriculture and Food were amalgamated. It was only because supplies were scarce that there was thought to be any need for a Ministry of Food. Again, there is no perceivable "health" basis for the decision to amalgamate. Winnifrith argues:

> On the grounds of administrative convenience and efficiency the arguments seemed all in favour of amalgamation....,rather than splitting its [the Ministry of Food's] work up between a number of departments...(Winnifrith;1962,p39).

The effect of amalgamation was to concentrate all the decision making procedures under one roof and to make differences of opinion an intra, rather than an inter-departmental affair. While it has always been maintained that consumer interests were carefully considered in pricing policy, the opportunities for consumer input were negligible.

Agriculture clearly represents a policy sector, with particular political relationships which are broadly consensual in character. The food processing industry, which in many respects is closely related to the "primary producers", is much more complex in its structure of representation and production.

In the politics of dietary change, agricultural production and the National Farmers Union are key variables. Changes in the consumption of eggs, dairy products and meat would have large knock-on effects on the whole of agricultural production - witness the position of egg producers after the Salmonella in eggs scare. Equally, the fact that the position of the NFU is institutionalised within MAFF affords them access to decision making centres which could forestall attempts at dietary change either from within MAFF or the DoH.

It is important, therefore, to conceptualise these relationships. I would follow Smith (1988,1989) in arguing that the relations between the NFU and MAFF are best described as a *policy community*, that is, a pattern of relationships which are exclusive, integrated, have uneven resources, a consensus on policy values, and a particular field of authority and responsibility. There is an obvious, shared value system which revolves around continued state support for an expanding or protected agricultural sector. There are mutual benefits to both sides of the relationship, because of the financial rewards to farmers and the simplicity that NFU "hegemony" (Wilson;1977,p33) offers MAFF in consultations. Equally, despite the political advantages of the NFU it is clear that, in the last instance, the relations are asymmetric; that is, the state will impose solutions to problems if necessary. The structure of agriculture policy making suggests the exclusion of genuine consumer and professional interests, and their accommodation both within other networks which surround agriculture (particularly the technocratic network) and those networks built up around specific issues such as food labelling.

The fact that this value system imposes very great structural constraints, even upon an industry as powerful as food, suggests that agricultural interests are dominant in their own sector, and predominant over other sectors as well. This does not mean that the NFU have not been under considerable pressure over the past ten years to respond more directly to market mechanisms, it simply means that the arrangements for agriculture are predominant within MAFF.

Food Processing and Retailing

So far, it should be clear that much of the ideological and economic culture within MAFF comes from the perceptions of what its own role has been. This appears to be epitomised by the relationship between MAFF and the NFU.

Yet, it has consistently been argued that it is the food industry, rather than the farmers, who have exerted pressure on MAFF as far as dietary change is concerned (see for example Walker and Cannon;1985, Cannon;1987, National Forum;1988, Turner;1983b). This is complicated by the fact that Grant, for example, has argued that it is very difficult to talk of there being "a" food industry, when food processing encompasses such a wide range of products and interests (Grant;1983,p3-4).

As a hypothesis, the idea that food processors have exerted pressure on MAFF to contain the diet and health debate is plausible. Changes in compositional standards would affect them, not farmers. Changes to food labels would increase their costs and unfavourable information on those products could reduce sales. This hypothesis will be tested when we look at the government's response to the COMA report in Chapter Seven. For now, I simply want to look at how relations between MAFF and industry have developed and how we can characterise them.

Politically, the food industry has never enjoyed the institutionalised access to MAFF of the NFU. Its access to, and influence over, decision making has been far more informal, and in many ways, more intangible. While it is clear that the farmers have experienced a great many changing pressures, particularly over the past twenty years, the food industry has under-gone a transformation both structurally and with respect to its power with regard to other sections of the food chain.

These changes have manifested themselves politically although in the immediate post war period it appears that little had changed from war-time. Winnifrith wrote:

> The extent to which the Food Trades worked in or with
> the Ministry of Food was another wartime development
> with a peacetime sequel. When such men went back to

their old firms after the war, it was only natural that they and their old department should keep in touch with one another thus helping to preserve greater mutual understanding between the Government and the food industry (Winnifrith;1962,p37).

This should be seen in the context of the changing administrative arrangements for food and the creation of MAFF. Even though the farmers had captured a place for themselves in agricultural decision making, the food industry were largely unable to do the same in connection with those policies which affected them - food labelling and compositional standards. Cannon, for example, cites the Food Standards Committee's decision to reject a number of widely used food additives on health grounds in the 1950's (Cannon;1987,p178-184). This rejection was accepted by MAFF but challenged strongly by industry until many of them were wholly, or partly reinstated. This process took some twenty five years in all. Cannon drew the conclusion that the failure of industry to secure its preferred policy outcomes demonstrates the relative political weakness of the industry at the time.

Institutionally, the developing links between industry and MAFF were, with the exception of the meat and dairy sectors, largely informal. The meat and dairy sectors were both manufacturing and producing sectors, these had their own commodity divisions within MAFF and also had other institutions attached to them. In the case of milk and milk products, the Milk Marketing Board and what was, in 1979, to become the Dairy Trade Federation, virtually controlled all aspects of the purchase and distribution of milk. Of necessity there was a strong state involvement in this because until 1984 the state retained the option of setting a maximum price for liquid milk sales (Hollingham and Howarth;1989,p3 and 47-50). The success of the Milk Marketing Scheme for milk producers, prompted the NFU to urge MAFF to adopt a similar scheme for livestock. This was refused (consistently), but a concession was made in the form of the Meat and Livestock Commission (1967). The rest of the industry had to be content with being subsumed under what is now called Food Policy 1 Division.

But while industry may have access to MAFF, there are many aspects of policies which affect industry which they have very little say over. Of these, the Common Agricultural Policy (CAP) is the most painful. Until British entry into the EEC (1973), the method of agricultural subsidy was beneficial to farmers, food manufacturers and to consumers as well and, as such, contributed to the post war consensus that agricultural subsidy and expansion was generally desirable.

The system of price and market guarantees which operated until 1953 meant that it was the Exchequer which paid farmers through taxation. Consequently, prices to consumers and manufacturers were kept lower, and the costs of the subsidies were distributed progressively through the tax system itself. The deficiency payments scheme, which made up the deficiency between a set price and the market price, and which applied in various incarnations between 1953 and 1973, had the same effect on food processors.

This changed after Britain joined the EEC where "intervention" buying and import levies applied. Intervention buying occurs when the market price of a product falls below a pre-set Commission price; at this point, farmers may sell to intervention (the Commission). When this system has to operate it reduces market supply and raises prices to both consumers and manufacturers. Import levies, which are supposed to protect EEC producers, artificially raise the price of certain foods imported from non-EEC countries and, again, increase the costs to industry. Unsurprisingly, this has not gone un-noticed in the industry which views the CAP :

> ...as one of the major constraints within which it operates...A food processing company...has little influence over the price or indeed the nature of its raw material supplies originating in the EC (ACARD; 1982, p22, quoted in, Grant;1983,p24).

Thus from there being a broad consensus between manufacturers and producers on the type of state intervention that was desirable, and a reasonably coherent distinction between their policy interests, entry into the EEC politicised much of what had previously been taken as given.

Politically, a distinct ideological difference can be discerned between the two sides of the farm gate. During and after WWII the state (MAFF) came to accept an interventionist role in production for strategic and economic reasons but has shown a marked reluctance to intervene directly in the market place itself. Hence, food manufacturers operated under a different set of political constraints. Jupe, a MAFF official, has observed:

> Their [Ministers] general policy is that people should be left free to produce or to buy whatever they want, provided that everybody knows what it is (Jupe;

1985,p6).

He goes on to say that a consequence of this principle has been that: "..generally speaking British Ministers are not in favour of anything more than the absolute minimum of controls on the composition of food (Jupe;1985,p6)". This position is entirely consistent with the perceptions of the role of the market place in food supply I outlined earlier. In other words, the state has felt compelled to intervene substantially in production, but has steered well clear of extending that intervention into the market place. Ideologically, there is a strong and mutual interest between food manufacturers (and retailers) and MAFF in the preservation of a market place free from state interference. Of course, such a position does cause problems for dietary change. There is no doubt that if the state is going to have any role in promoting dietary change then it will, to a greater or lesser extent, impinge upon the free operation of the market. The fact that the relationship between MAFF and the food industry is predicated upon minimalist interference is therefore extremely important.

This does not, of course, imply that manufactured products go unregulated; it has been argued that: "More law bears down on food manufacturers than any other single sector of manufacturing industry (Turner;1981,p19, quoted in, Grant;1983,p21)". During the post war period the general legislation controlling food composition and labelling, which began with the Food Act of 1875, has been extended. In 1953 for example, a full list of ingredients were required on all products and by 1967 certain additives had to be listed. The regulation of the industry serves two purposes. Its primary purpose, of course, is to protect or inform the consumer but regulations also legitimise the goods that are offered for sale. It is this legitimising role which makes regulations more welcome to industry than you might expect:

> Manufacturers say they dislike regulations. Compositional regulations in particular are criticised on the ground that they inhibit innovation. But in fact regulation is surprisingly popular. Businessmen master regulations very rapidly and thoroughly in a way that impresses Civil Servants and seem to use them as reference points in running their business (Jupe; 1985,p5).

Regulations, or any other type of state intervention in the market are welcomed *as long as they do not interfere with the competitiveness of the firms in that market*. Again, we return to the idea that the rules of the game between MAFF and industry preserve industry's right to compete fairly in the market. This qualification can take many forms. For example, the selective food subsidies on butter, tea, sugar and bread of 1974 were condemned by the then FMF (Food Manufacturers Federation) because it was thought that they gave a competitive advantage to the producers of those products that were subsidised. Similarly, regulations which are thought unduly restrictive will be challenged because they affect the ability of firms to innovate and to stay competitive. Restrictions which raise the costs of products are also unwelcome.

It is not difficult to see, therefore, that the Common Agricultural Policy would be seen as an unnecessary interference in the workings of the market. Despite the many cleavages within the industry which promote conflicts between, for example, those who freeze food and those that "can" food, the principle of a free market is a strong unifying force within the industry as a whole. This suggests that the political homogeneity of food manufacturers should be seen on two levels.

At the empirical level, the fact that the industry produces 50,000 different products (FDF;undated,p2) and can be easily divided into relatively autonomous product sectors indicates a diverse and, by implication, weakened food industry. However, there is another, ideological, level at which there is a great deal of agreement between the food sectors on how they should compete with each other and what the role of the state should be. In Chapter Seven, for example, I will argue that the present government has consistently looked towards the operation of the market, and consumer sovereignty in particular, to promote dietary changes. Such a position is, of course, consistent with a predisposition of the state not to get involved in the market.

This ideological compatibility suggests that between MAFF and the food industry generally there is a great deal of common ground, both in their perceptions of each others roles and in their orientation to public policy. One observer has described this relationship as "soft corruption" because policies invariably consider the competitiveness of industry over and above consumer interests. For example, in 1980, the Food Standards Committee (FSC) of MAFF recommended that the regulations governing meat products should be tightened because consumers were not aware that water was being added to products, or that the definition of meat did not refer simply to lean meat (Food Standards Committee;1980). The subsequent regulations (MAFF;1984) did not require the *lean* content of meat to be labelled nor did they stop the practice of adding weight to a product by injecting water. In interview, a representative of the meat industry said that the regulations represented a compromise between the interests of consumers and industry (Personal Correspondence (H);1987). He argued that his organisation had not got things all its own way, although he appeared not to realise that the regulations were some distance from the recommendations contained in the FSC report. In short, the ideological compatibility means that regardless of whether industry has to argue over the details of policy with MAFF, the parameters within which eventual policies will fall are already agreed - they are part of the rules of the game.

But the political influence of industry extends beyond this ideological compatibility with the state. Besides the access that industry has to decision making structures, it is increasingly the case that politically sensitive decisions are actually being made by the representatives of industry.

In 1982 an ACARD[1] report recommended that the government set up and sponsor committees to guide research and development within the food industry (ACARD;1982) and this call was echoed in a NEDC report (NEDC;1986). These committees have now been established and each is Chaired by a representative of industry. Similarly, the present government has made it known that the food research that it funds will be more market-orientated than before, and that once the market potential of the research is clear, industry will be expected to take it over (The Food Programme;1989).

Even the standing committees which advise MAFF have been criticised because many of their members come from industry. It has been difficult conclusively to establish that industry has been influential in their decisions because the proceedings of these committees are covered by the Official Secrets Act. In the past it has been the Food Standards Committee (FSC) and the Food Additives and Contaminants Committee (FACC) which have advised MAFF on those aspects of policy which are of concern to us. Neither of these bodies were statutory and MAFF was not bound by their recommendations. They have now been amalgamated to form the Food Advisory Committee (FAC), the title of which leaves few doubts as to its role in policy making. The membership of these committees always shows a strong industry presence. For example, of the twelve members of the FAC in 1987 four came from industry (Feedback;1987,p3). Cannon, in a thorough survey of the membership of 19 MAFF committees concluded that nearly half the members had had links with industry, although this included

---

[1] Advisory Council for Applied Research and Development.

those academics who had been sponsored by industry in their research. The same was true of DoH committees as well (Cannon;1987,p314).

The conclusions that can be drawn from knowing the membership of these committees are limited without further knowing what was said during committee meetings. However, it is possible to infer from other examples what the orientation of "technocrats" may be. There is a strong degree of cross membership between MAFF committees, the Scientific and Technical Committee of the Food and Drink Federation (FDF) and the industry-sponsored British Nutrition Foundation (BNF). Again, Cannon (1987;p135-137) was given the proceedings of a BNF committee which was considering a publication on sugar. The minutes suggested that both the scientific and commercial implications of changes in sugar consumption would be considered in the final draft of the report.

The degree of influence that industry can exert over public policy belies their seemingly limited institutional incorporation. The industry has an automatic right to consultation which it shares with consumer groups. However, unlike consumer groups, the industry shares with MAFF an ideological orientation toward policy which consistently tends to maintain the position of industry at the expense of the consumer. This is perhaps the greatest consequence of "sponsorship". Despite the fact that the dominating policy community of the farmers and MAFF exerts a great deal of structural influence over food manufacturers it appears that, within this constraint, food manufacturers have a niche of their own which provides them with policy latitude. Before we try to conceptualise the relationships within MAFF I want to return to what I called the "transformation" of the food manufacturing industry since WWII.

This "transformation" did not refer to its political relationships, but to the structure of the industry and the balance of power within the food chain. Without some knowledge of the commercial context within which the industry is operating it is difficult to fully understand the motives and actions of the industry.

Transformation The food manufacturing sector, like many other areas of manufacturing, has experienced a great deal of amalgamation and diversification over the past twenty years or so. This has tended to concentrate productive power in fewer and fewer hands (Hardman;1986,p37). The commercial pressure on the industry generally has come from similar structural changes in the food retailing sector, rather than from competition within manufacturing. The top six food retailers now control some 52% of all grocery sales (Grant;1983,p13) and have extended the concentration in the sector which began in the inter-war period. With so few customers controlling such a high percentage of total sales, manufacturers have often been forced to sell at very reduced profit margins to their larger customers (Swinbank, Burns and Beard;1985,p3). Most of the larger retailers produce their own-name products which are often sub-contracted out to brand-name producers, and which under-cut the price of brand name products. So, retail concentration and own-name products both reinforce the predominance of retailers and undermine the autonomy of manufacturers to innovate and compete openly in the market. In interview, a retailing executive said that his company had no qualms about demanding product changes from their suppliers, even in the manufacturer's brand-name products (Personal Correspondence (P);1986).

The extent to which this has affected manufacturers can be seen from a Monopolies and Mergers Commission report conceived to look into the practice of "Discounts to Retailers" (MMC;1981). This report dealt with other manufacturing industries as well, and concluded that the practice of retailers demanding these discounts was not against the public interest. There was also a report from the Office of Fair Trading (OFT) on the same subject which came to the same conclusion (OFT;1985).

In addition, the food industry generally has been faced with fairly low profit rates and, of course, did not escape the recession of the early 1980's (NEDC;1986,p1-2). The response of the industry, unsurprisingly, has been to look for new products to sell and these tend to fall into three broad categories; health, convenience, and luxury foods (NEDC;1986,p4). The simultaneous growth of these product ranges, which appear to be contradictory in many respects, reflects the commercial position that industry finds itself in and, of course, underlines the reason why it believes it must be free to innovate - so they may respond to commercial incentives. An executive from Tesco's, which has been highly praised for its healthy eating policy, has said:

> ...we recognised two types of opportunity, firstly to provide our customers with a service they wanted and secondly to benefit from significant amounts of potentially favourable publicity (Mason;1985,p8).

The same may be said of the FDF's decision to co-fund with MAFF a food intolerance data-bank (Feedback;1987,p1). This has not been done for reasons of public health, but because it may help allay public fears about the composition of foods.

Obviously enough, it is the market position of the food industry which determines much of what it does. While it is not in the industry's interests to have severe and adverse health effects from food consumption, it is MAFF's responsibility to ensure that this does not happen, not industry's. Manufacturers and retailers will respond to the market, and cannot be meaningfully assigned any degree of public-spiritedness which threatens their commercial viability.

We now have the basis for conceptualising these relationships theoretically. Beneath the over-arching policy community of agriculture there are a series of political networks which are functional and relate to certain food policy needs. Some of these networks are centred on product areas (such as meat and dairy products). These networks are not easily distinguished from one another because there is much cross membership, for example, the Dairy Trade Federation belongs to a policy community controlling milk sales but also to a network interested in food labelling. The term "producer network" is useful to the extent that it can label these networks and draw our attention to things which the members have in common. For our purposes we are particularly interested in the market orientation of network members because this appears to be an axial principle of the relationship between food manufacturers and MAFF. Equally, though sub-sectors such as milk and meat behave more like policy communities with a limited membership and less market orientation.

The technocratic element is pervasive as it encompasses not only MAFF officials but also elements of the peak organisations (the FDF) and the advisory committees; indeed, it stretches to the DoH as well. Under these circumstances it is reasonable to see this a network in its own right. The impression, then, is not of a fixed institutional arrangement, unless policies are strongly linked to agriculture. Rather, there are numerous networks formulating around issues which may or may not recur, operating within known rules of the game but on an ad hoc basis. The membership of many of these networks may not be consistent across issues but members will always enter the network on the understanding that rules do apply.

A Post-War Nutrition Policy?

Despite the fact that MAFF has a fairly narrow conception of its health responsibilities, it is still possible to argue that Britain has enjoyed a nutrition policy in the post-WWII period. If this is so, does it represent a means of implementing the dietary changes recommended for reducing heart disease, or indeed, for changing other aspects of diet such as sugar, salt and fibre consumption?

Darke (1979) has argued that Britain has had a nutrition policy and her argument is convincing, though ultimately unconsoling. The crux of the argument rests with what the nutritional problems of the pre-war period were thought to be, in short, these were problems of price and availability. It is not difficult to imagine that a policy of production maximisation might be consistent with this, because it would tend to lower the price of food. Darke outlines the logic behind the post-war policy:

> The welfare state and National Health Service were set up. Government was responsible for a nutritious food supply which was toxocologically and micro-biologically safe. Food subsidies ensured that staple foods were within the purchasing power of all. A social security system made provision for any who were disadvantaged either through ill-health or economically. The Welfare Food Scheme continued to provide milk and vitamin supplements for expectant mothers and young children. The Milk in Schools scheme provided free of charge 1/3 pint of milk on each school day for all school children. A mid-day meal was available at school for any who wished to have it and was free of charge to the impoverished. Medicine and medical treatment were available to all (Darke; 1979,p40-41).

There are a number of points that should be drawn out from this. Firstly, malnutrition is still seen as a function of deprivation, hence the references to the social security system and the welfare state. Again, this suggests that post-war policy was, quite rightly, influenced by the problems that had existed before the war. Secondly, there is a clear distinction made between the population in general, and those "vulnerable" groups within the population. The vulnerable groups are defined as those who are either physically or financially unable to support themselves nutritionally and so need assistance.

Prevention and Health (DHSS;1977) argues for a distinction to be made between a "food policy" which "ensures that sufficient safe and wholesome food is made available to the public." (DHSS;1977,p42) and a "nutrition policy" which includes research, advice, information and "action to see that nutritional needs are met." (DHSS;1977,p42). Once again, the health and food aspects of the policies are conceptually and institutionally separated. The "safe and wholesome" supply is the responsibility of MAFF and operates at the population level, while the "nutrition policy" which lies with the Department of Health (DoH) emphasises the vulnerable sections of the population. This is an oversimplification to the extent that health obviously does figure in the calculations of MAFF. Jupe has said:

> Leaving aside ...the subject of health risk caused by bad dietary habits, the safety issues which face Government are essentially controlling the use of additives and preventing contamination (Jupe;1985,p2).

The point is that the safety of the diet is a DoH responsibility; the safety of the foods that constitute the diets are split between MAFF (eg.the Food Advisory Committee) and the DoH (eg. the Committee on the Medical Aspects of Chemicals in Food and the Environment). Officially it is the DoH who advises MAFF and its expert committees but, in reality, there is plenty of expertise within MAFF anyway.

The distinction between the responsibilities of the departments is also oversimplified to the extent that not all DoH interest in nutrition is confined to vulnerable groups. It is, for example, responsible for advising on the Recommended Daily Amounts (RDA's) of vitamins and minerals to the population. However, intervention is *largely* directed at the vulnerable and that this has historically been the accepted position within the DoH and between the DoH and MAFF. Again, this amounts to a manifest reluctance to intervene on the demand side of food:

> In connection with diet the role of Government is directed primarily towards assembling, assessing and disseminating information, based on scientific evidence, in the light of which individuals can form their own views and take their own decisions (DHSS;1977,p40).

Even the best efforts of state agencies to provide food which was cheap, plentiful, safe and wholesome still did not get around the problem that the safety net of welfare intervention was still necessary, and remains so.

But such a division of responsibility is based upon certain assumptions about the nature of the food supply. Firstly, it assumes that the food on offer in the market (to those who are not vulnerable) is nutritionally adequate and/or desirable. If the problems before the war were of undernourishment and if it was believed that a balanced diet would provide all the nutrients essential to health, then the policy outlined above is entirely consistent. Consumers need only the means to purchase a varied and balanced diet, and the problems of undernourishment have been solved. If, on the other hand, nutritional wisdom changes, as it did by degrees in the 1970's, then this is not necessarily the case. If the balance of the food supply is such that the food itself (rather than the lack of it) becomes the problem then simply consuming a variety of what is available will not ensure a person's health. A further implication is that simply encouraging farmers to produce as much as possible, or limiting their production for reasons other than health, will also be insufficient because it cannot ensure the correct balance within the food chain as a whole.

Given this, our nutrition policy does not appear to suggest that it provides a strong basis for professional influence. Such influence has not extended into MAFF because it has concentrated on the vulnerable, a group which by and large can be dealt with without reference to MAFF. Thus, while food safety is a concern of MAFF, nutrition has never been a major input into its policies.

If health professionals propose that the balance of the food chain be altered by, for example, reducing its fat content, then this in turn implies that MAFF's traditional regard for the competitiveness of the food sector may be questioned. Lastly, while the state has been willing to protect, advise and supply the vulnerable, the success of post-war policies has meant that it has seldom been necessary for the state to direct the consumption patterns of the whole population. Where advice has been available, for example, through MAFF's *Manual of Nutrition*, the information has been uncontentious, and has reflected the nutritional orthodoxy of the post-war period.

Since WWII, agricultural production and policies relating to food have been taken as given, and the health and nutritional aspects of food have simply "mopped up" the shortcomings of the market and MAFF. Thus the dominant political influences over the food supply have emanated both ideologically and institutionally from MAFF and the DoH has played an advisory and complementary role. This system relies upon most of the population, most of the time, believing that they do not suffer diet-related health problems. If such problems are perceived to exist then the system of food supply is called into question. This is precisely what has happened in the 1970's and the 1980's, and it was accompanied by recommendations, such as those from health professionals, for a return to a more highly integrated food and nutrition policy.

Conclusion

A number of the major themes established in the previous chapter still hold true after WWII. Notable amongst these has been the states pre-disposition to retain, as far as possible, the competitveness and innovativeness of industry. This much, perhaps, is only to be expected, but in conjunction with state support for agriculture these arrangements elevate the importance of MAFF with regard to dietary policies. Many of the decisions which affect the health of the population are food and agriculture decisions, as opposed to health decisions. This makes the way in which decisions are made within MAFF very important.

The aim of this chapter has been twofold. Firstly, I hope to have demonstrated the closed nature of policy within MAFF. Secondly, I hope that the basis of policy are clear. These are important because jointly they infer that any attempts at dietary change will have to have the consent of MAFF, but also that the new policies will have to be consistent with the old. What Darke has called Britain's post-war nutrition policy fits the bill very nicely because it impinges very little on food and agriculture policies, but rather, concentrates on the vulnerable sections of the population. Consequently, it does not really provide a good test of how successful attempts at dietary change at the population level will be.

Another way of testing this would be to explore the power and the role of health professionals. As yet we have not discussed these, and it could be that despite their lack of institutional involvement, they are powerful enough to force through dietary change. This is the subject of the following chapter.

6 Health and Prevention Since WWII

Chapter Two suggested that the power of professionals may well have been over-estimated, particularly when they are placed in a broad political context. As major agents in the politics of dietary change, their role is going to be important, but this still leaves the problem of establishing where, why and how they may be powerful. Equally, it may also suggest reasons why health professionals, elite or otherwise, might be less interested in preventing CHD than we might expect.

There are other reasons why "health" in general might be important. The role of preventive medicine or the existing policies to combat CHD will both give some indication of how well dietary change might be incorporated into policies which already exist. Once again, we return to the question of how likely dietary change is, given the policies and structures that we have at the moment?

This chapter is going to give a very general overview of the nature of professional power in Britain, the orientation of the health care system and the role of preventive medicine.

With current government reforms still underway it is difficult to establish conclusively how these reforms will affect professionals within the NHS.

For our purposes, this is perhaps less important than might be expected for although change is inevitable, we are primarily interested in the period up to 1984 - before the present reforms came in.

The central points which will be made are; where health professionals have been seen as powerful, this has relied upon their position within the NHS and the power they can wield there; the unitary, centralised nature of the NHS makes innovation less likely than in other, decentralised systems; an emphasis on curative medicine and the problems of preventive medicine both militate against dietary change being given a high priority by health professionals.

The Health Service and Health Professionals

Since 1948, Britain has had a unitary system of health-care provision funded by the state. The 1946 Act effectively nationalised voluntary and local authority hospitals. The primary sector, including general practice, was administratively separate, with GP's remaining self employed. From the beginning, there were administrative problems both because the "tripartite" structure has separated the various branches of the services, and because the NHS has had an apparently limitless capacity to increase its expenditure.

Both the reorganisations of the service (1974 and 1980) were attempts to enhance the administrative efficiency of the service; in 1974, by integrating the acute hospital sector more fully with the rest of the community services and, in 1982, by removing completely one of the administrative tiers (Area Health Authorities). Integrating the service by making it both more cost effective and responsive to centrally prescribed goals has been seen as a means to curb increasing costs and of achieving greater uniformity in the services provided across Britain.

During the 1970's it was believed that planning the service centrally would be the answer to these problems. The difficulties of planning for the health needs of the population when the administration of the service was "discontinuous" (Wistow;1989,p3) were manifest:

> It is hard to escape the conclusion that the structure of
> the NHS, particularly the relationship between the
> DHSS and the regions and the regions and the DHSS,
> has contributed to the inability of the health services to

111

allocate resources fairly and rationally on the basis of overall health needs (Owen;1976,p8).

This amounts to a structural problem which detracts from there being a single vision of what the goals of the NHS might be. It has been difficult, therefore, either to dictate from the centre what the periphery should be doing, or for the periphery to pursue unified and consistent goals across the country.

Historically, the central department funding the NHS has kept a discreet distance from the running of the service. As Harrison has argued: "In the period from 1948 to about 1982, governments have had little real interest in control of doctors by NHS managers (1988,p22)".

This does not mean that the centre has been insensitive or unconcerned about the running of the service, but rather, that it accepted that there were limits to how far it could direct the service from above through the use of managers. The Regional, District and/or Area Health Authorities have been administered by boards which have been dominated by professionals. As a consequence of this, it has often been the case that the wishes of central government have been frustrated by professional control of the bureaucracy of the NHS: "In the NHS, the agenda, especially at local level, has been controlled by the medical profession (Haywood and Alaszewski; 1980,p136)". Even the present government's early re-organisation, which allowed for politically appointed Regional and District Chairs and the introduction of managerialism, appears not to have made much difference to the balance of forces in the periphery. Ham has argued:"...there [is] little evidence...of any change in the balance of power in the NHS (Ham;1986,p129)." This point is also made by Harrison (1988). It is wrong to assume, however, that this situation has been accepted by Ministers of Health as either inevitable, or necessarily desirable. The 1983 Griffiths Report (DHSS;1983) provided the basis for the introduction of managerialism into the health service and the recent white paper *Working for Patients* (DHSS;1988) is a step towards the corporatisation of health care. The extent to which professionals retain their former predominant position within the NHS after the changes in 1991 remains to be seen although there is evidence to suggest that managerialism and budgeting within hospitals also provides health professionals with opportunities to circumvent some of the new constraints upon them. Having said this, it is also true that the strategic decision making at district and regional level can no longer be done by professionals who command a majority on these authorities. From our point of view, we are concerned primarily with the nature of the system and sources of professional power, real or otherwise. I will deal with each of these in turn.

The experiences of the 1970's, when successive governments attempted to re-orientate the NHS and set its own priorities (DHSS;1976) (at the expense of the acute sector) suggests that regardless of the wishes of central government, professionals had the ability to maintain their own priorities. Wistow(1989), gives the example of the "Cinderella services" (those for the elderly and the mentally ill and handicapped) which were supposed to benefit from the redirection of resources away from acute medicine. This was opposed by health professionals both officially, in that original target savings were significantly revised after professional protestation, and unofficially where the implementation of policy was frustrated locally. Haywood and Alaszewski, for example, cite the case of money forwarded to Regional Health Authorities for "secure units" for violent or difficult patients. Three years after the money had been allocated, four regions had not even devised plans for the units, none had been opened, and the £5m had been absorbed into the regional budgets for other purposes (1980,p49). A similar example comes from the 1962 Hospital Plan that all districts should be served with a District General Hospital (DGH). Even here, many of the hospitals were greatly influenced by the demands of professionals, which tended to make them larger than had originally been planned (Klein;1983,p73-75). Ham (1981), in his study of health authorities in Leeds, characterises this type of decision making as working within a "dominant incrementalist mode"; the processes are plural and "characterised by bargaining and compromise, the distribution of power was weighed heavily in favour of the professional monopolisers" (Ham;1981,p198).

A consequence of a unified system of health care provision and a well-integrated professional representation is that it tends to make the British profession more "conservative" than, for example, the American system which is more disaggregated. Hollingsworth (1986), in a comparison between the British and the American systems of health care, concluded that:

> Across countries, centralised systems have been less costly in financial terms, but they have tended to be less innovative, especially technical innovations, which are very costly. There has been much literature that indicates that centralisation has stifled the adoption of new ideas and slowed down the process of

communication.

He argues that the reasons for this are:

> ...the exclusion of particular interest groups from the
> decision making process, the reliance on public funding,
> and the avoidance of specialised services have made
> certain types of innovation appear more costly and
> unnecessary (Hollingsworth;1986,p248-249).

There are two points which should be made here. The first is that if
Hollingsworth is correct in asserting that "centralised" systems are less
likely to adopt new ideas, then this would go some way to explaining why
the British medical profession have appeared more reluctant to accept the
evidence on diet and health than their counterparts in other countries. The
other point is that the response from the centre to these "new" ideas would,
as Hollingsworth notes, be considered at the aggregate level, that is, how
the ideas afect the whole service. The cost implications of such policies,
therefore, may play a much greater part in decisions that were made
because they are being made at the system level rather than the local level.

It seems clear that the ability of health professionals to exert influence on
health issues differed markedly depending on whether the solution to the
issues resided inside or outside of the NHS. Within the NHS, there exists a
"professionalised network" and policy communities which determined
much of the level and direction of expenditure, and maintained existing
priorities, which were primarily curative in nature. This network is
functionally constructed in that the resources accumulated and protected by
the professionals (Freidson, 1970) are those necessary for them to retain
their autonomy and professional status. On the other hand health issues
which are marginal to the predominantly curative ideology, and to the
calculations and influence of professionals seemed less predictable. The
structure of the NHS has tended to predispose the system of health care to
maintain this type of direction, and the unitary character of the service also
tends to stifle the adoption of new ideas and innovations.

With regard to the politics of dietary change this is significant because it
suggests no necessary or compelling reason why health professionals should
be able to exert great influence over political decisions unless they have
procedural controls available to them or they can exercise clinical autonomy
over the implementation of policies.

What, then, are the sources of professional power within the NHS? It seems this power can be accounted for in three ways; the curative nature of western medicine in general; the ethos of clinical autonomy and administrative control over resource allocation. This last point has already been dealt with so I will concentrate on the other two.

The "curative" nature of western medicine has been criticised by many people. Dubos (1960), for example, makes the distinction between an ideology of "health restored" as opposed to one of "health preserved" (quoted in Wistow;1989). Illich, a strong critic of technocratic and technological intervention, holds similar views and is scathing about the role of professionals in actually causing ill-health:

> In rich countries the deaths caused by the use of evacuation equipment are beginning to balance the number of lives thus saved. Hospital "worship" is unrelated to the hospitals performance.
> Like any other growth industry, the health system directs its products where demand seems unlimited: into defence against death (Illich;1976,p112-113).

This ideology is as evident in Britain as it is anywhere else. The elite professionals are those that intervene and operate on the heart and the brain, not those that prevent cardiovascular diseases:

> Professional interest is increasingly absorbed by methods of investigation and treatment whose complexities seem to challenge the attention of the best minds and whose rewards are assumed to justify it (McKeown;1976,p136).

This type of care can become self perpetuating because it links in with another source of professional power which both Klein and Hunter recognise as the ability of professionals to pre-empt expenditure through innovation (Klein;1983, Hunter;1980). The basis of this type of argument is that the momentum generated by research and innovation in the NHS presents central government with a *fait accompli* in terms of resource allocation. Its other consequence is, of course, that it tends to work in favour of the status quo - a hi-tech', curative service will, on this analysis, remain so. This type of ideology not only favours existing institutions, but also colours perceptions of what a health service should be - a health service is one that cures illness rather than prevents it.

The ethos of clinical autonomy has also been institutionalised:

> whatever the organisation, the doctors taking part must
> remain free to direct their clinical knowledge and
> personal skill for the benefit of the patients in the way in
> which they feel to be best (MoH;1944. *quoted in*:
> Wistow;1989,p10).

This is perhaps the core principle from which other sources of professional power emanate. In Chapter Two (Theoretical Perspectives) it was argued that the power of professionals has been seen as residing in the client-practitioner relationship.   It is the ethos of clinical autonomy, the professional privilege to examine, diagnose and prescribe, which forms the basis of this relationship.   It also underpins the position of the professional within the NHS in general.   Recent studies to assess the impact of the "new managerialism" on the behaviour of professionals have found clinical autonomy remains largely unaffected:

> Clinical performance was "still regarded as professional
> territory or as one .... consultant put it, management
> stops at the consulting room door" (Harrison, Hunter,
> Marnock and Pollitt;1989,p5 *in* Wistow:1989,p18).

As Owen suggests however, "..many doctors began to see clinical freedom as a licence to ignore all considerations of cost and resources in the practice of clinical medicine (Owen;1976,p80)".   This is the crux of the conflict which now exists between the Thatcher government and the medical profession. It is not difficult to see how the principle of clinical autonomy has been institutionalised in, for example, their control over hospital plans and through the procedural controls in the health authorities.   There are numerous studies which suggest that their ability to influence and direct their work environment in accordance with their own wishes was unparalleled by virtually any other profession. All of these studies draw upon the fact that this influence was derived from one of the three sources mentioned above. Ham (1981,p198) for example, argues that within the NHS professional power comes from professional membership of Regional Hospital Boards and Hospital Management Boards, their presence on advisory committees, their position as service providers and the deference which is afforded them. My argument, therefore, is that commentators have looked towards the nature of the relationship between professionals and clients to measure the power of the profession and have seen additional evidence in the commanding position of professionals within the health service to support their contention. Whether such power will survive the present reforms is less important than the fact that this scenario does not necessarily imply an equally strong outside of the health care system.

It is not difficult to see, therefore, that Rhodes' characterisation of the health service as a "professionalised network" is largely accurate. There is a high degree of horizontal integration because of shared or similar tasks and a pervading ideology. Equally, there is little vertical articulation because of the decentralised nature of decision-making and the absence of strong accountability procedures. Similarly, Alford's (1975) distinction between professional monopolisers, corporate rationalisers (the new managerialism) and user/community interests (patients) is an equally useful characterisation of the contending interests which now exist within the NHS. This is entirely compatible with Rhodes' characterisation of a professionalised network.

For our purposes, however, this discussion of professional power is incomplete. So far, the focus has been upon the ability of professionals to influence their work environment, and this ability is clearly considerable. But not all health issues are germinated and resolved within the NHS and the "structure" of health care is necessarily broader than the pattern of relationships that constitute the NHS. Recent attempts (Griffiths;1988) to find a formula to integrate the health and social services testify that it is difficult to draw a neat dividing line between health and other issues.

The extent to which professionals can replicate their success within the operation of the NHS depends upon their ability to either extend their professionalised network into other arenas, or, to use their resources (knowledge, authority, autonomy etc.) to generate new resources which are useful to them.

This may not be as easy as it sounds. Klein observed that:

> When the stage widens to bring on the actors who normally play no part in the health care arena....when the Treasury and Cabinet become involved - then the ability of the medical profession to get its own way diminishes (Klein;1983,p56).

Even within the NHS, other resources can be brought to bear which dilute the influence of professionals. These are the broader economic and political constraints which were also recognised by Haywood and

Alaszewski. While it is true that professionals are dominant within the structure of the NHS, Haywood and Alaszewski argue that the centre has a strong "negative" power (1980,p13) in that it can place limits on the actions of the periphery even if it cannot direct those actions explicitly. It is the positive side of this power that the present government is attempting to develop now. So, the first qualification to the power of professionals is that in the broader political sense, health must contend for resources with, for example, defence, education, transport etc.

Equally, just because health professionals have considerable weight within the NHS does not mean that all health issues can be resolved within the NHS itself. Brand, for example, cites the case of water fluoridation in Scotland, which was delayed both because of the intricacies of water authority administration and because of a free vote in local councils (Brand;1971). Read (1989) argues that professionals have been conspicuously unable to break the relationships that exist between the tobacco industry and government departments which allow ineffectual warnings on cigarette packets, taxation increases below the rate of inflation etc. Similarly, Doyal and Epstein (1983) catalogue the health problems associated with a number of carciogenic substances used in industry which persist because of their commercial value. In all of these cases it can be argued that professionals have the ability to place issues on the political agenda, but have not been able to resolve them. The conceptual distinction needs to be made, therefore, between issues which can be dealt with primarily within the confines of the NHS, and those which cannot.

Finally, even if professionals are granted access to other decision making forums, as might be the case in expert committees, the resources that they are able to direct are primarily those which they bear themselves (eg. their knowledge). To this extent, the "advisory" role of these committees (for example, the Food Advisory Committee and the Committee on the Medical Aspects of Food Policy) indicates that the clinical autonomy of professionals under these circumstances extends only to their judgements, not the practice of that autonomy. The terms of their engagement are therefore re-defined once they leave their place of work.

A qualification which may have to be made to this comes from how far preventive medicine has become institutionalised in Britain or has complemented the obvious curative bias in the NHS. If prevention were pervasive it may be possible to argue that professional resources were less necessary because complementary and compatible preventive measures were well established and had a momentum of their own.

> Everybody will agree that, of the two types of
> knowledge [curative and preventive], that which leads to
> the eradication of disease is the much more important to
> the community" (MRC;1937, in, Landsborough-
> Thomson;1975,p73).

During the 1970's, the ethos of prevention gained much ground in Britain
and elsewhere, notably Canada. Its political utility is that it may help solve
the endemic problem of NHS costs and, of course, save lives. But
prevention has been seen as an opportunity to place the weight of
responsibility for preventing ill-health upon the individuals themselves.
Indeed, there are many areas in which this financial utility is not at all
obvious anyway. Prevention, as defined by the DHSS (1977) is:

> ...either an attempt to prevent disease or disability
> before it occurs (primary prevention), the early
> detection and treatment of conditions with a view to
> returning the patient to normal health (secondary
> prevention), or the continuing treatment of disease or
> disability to avoid needless progression or complications
> (tertiary prevention) (DHSS;1977,p82).

As a working definition this is largely unhelpful. Many things which
intuitively might be regarded as curative, such as the treatment of
degenerative diseases, are, in fact defined as preventive; in this case,
preventing death, rather than preventing illness in the first place. Acheson
makes a similar point when he argues that tertiary prevention is not actually
prevention at all, but treatment (Acheson;1988,p174). It is little wonder,
therefore, that the DHSS could confidently assert that: "The Government
believes that a meaningful estimate of the total sum spent on prevention
cannot be achieved..... (DHSS;1977,p3)". The DHSS were responding to a
report by a Sub-Committee of the Expenditure Committee of the House of
Commons, which had argued that there should be a redistribution of
available resources in favour of preventive services and away from the
acute sector.

For our purposes, it is primary and secondary prevention which are the
most important. The primary approach is where prevention of heart disease
might occur; the secondary is where it might be detected. These

correspond to the "population" approach, and the "high risk" approach outlined in Chapter Three.

Contrary to the assertion made by the DHSS in 1977, The Committee of Public Accounts accepted that expenditure on prevention within the NHS could be estimated at around £600m in 1986 (Committee of Public Accounts;1986,i). As the DHSS had recognised, however, even within the category of prevention some aspects fall within the remit of the NHS and others do not. There is a very large difference between the levels of expenditure when they include public health measures (such as clean air and sewage treatment) and when they do not.

The scope of prevention can, therefore, be extremely broad. As with other aspects of the work of the DoH, much that is classified as preventive is concerned with the vulnerable sections of the population. For example, the immunisation of children, the school doctor service, health visiting and the like.

Given that not all "preventive" health measures are the responsibility of the DoH, where has the DoH seen its role as being? Allsop has argued:

> The role of government is seen to be primarily
> concerned with encouraging healthier lifestyles through
> providing information, and funding health education and
> health promotion (Allsop;1984,p178).

This is borne out by the *Prevention and Health* White Paper in which the DHSS replied to the 58 recommendations of the Sub-Committee's report. Health education, research and health promotion are generally seen as valid and acceptable policy options to pursue. The DHSS showed more reluctance to commit itself if (1) commercial interests are involved, in this case, the tobacco, drinks and food industries, or (2) the structure or resources of the NHS are likely to change, for example, reallocating resources away from high-technology toward prevention, and establishing a fund to train Health Visitors.

This can be explained by two things. Firstly, the ideology of lifestyle intervention has been one of providing people with information to make decisions for themselves. Health promotion and education fit very neatly into this ideology and can be administered largely within the structure of the NHS or related agencies (eg. the Health Education Authority).

Secondly, the reluctance of the DHSS to interfere with commercial interests reflects both the definition of health care which operates within the health care system (ie. to cure rather than to prevent), and the specific responsibilities of the DoH which are confined largely to the NHS itself. Similarly, Navarro has argued:

> ...the overall priority given to property and capital accumulation explains why, when health and property conflict, the latter usually takes priority over the former (Navarro;1976,p163,*in*, Black et al;1984).

While this is not necessarily a deterministic relationship, nevertheless, the role of capital does place a structural constraint upon the actions of the state, and the DoH. This is not to say that high rates of heart disease are in the interests of capital, but rather, that moves to reduce that level may not be.

This, then, is one constraint under which primary prevention may have to operate - that the message of prevention or the actions of the state may be curtailed by structural economic considerations. But the questions of costs in general have been central to successive governments' considerations of what preventive strategies to employ:

> Prevention is better than cure - but is it also cheaper?....Where, by relatively inexpensive means we can avoid condemning someone to a lifetime of physical dependence the answer will almost certainly be "yes"....But it would be foolish not to recognise that the advantages of prevention must be purchased at the cost of other services (DHSS;1976a,p84).

Prevention and Health:Everybody's Business (1976a) identifies some of the areas in which prevention is cheaper than cure (immunisation and vaccination) and those where it may not be (screening for breast cancer and Downs Syndrome for example).

On this basis, the predisposition to favour health education, information and health promotion is entirely understandable, because it is a relatively cheap form of prevention. (The budget for the Health Education Council (HEC) in 1985 was approximately £10m.)

The 1974 reorganisation of the NHS was supposed to simplify the arrangements for health education:

> Within the improved administrative framework of the reorganised NHS it is now possible for the first time to

undertake comprehensive planning and co-ordination of national and local policies and priorities (DHSS; 1977,p8).

As Allsop has argued, however, the structure of the agencies responsible for health education in Britain were such as to make a consistent and comprehensive strategy difficult to achieve:

> The lack of clear responsibility for community and environmental health at local level is mirrored by the lack of single departmental responsibility at central government level (Allsop;1984,p186-187).

This was indeed the case; there are Primary Health Care Teams consisting of GPs, Health Visitors and District Nurses; Health Education Officers who may be employed either by Health Authorities or Local Authorities; District Community Physicians to monitor services and Clinical Medical Officers who operate with schools. The Health Education Council, which was created in 1968, replaced a national organisation run and financed by local authorities. It was always seriously under-funded in relation to the job it had to do and was criticised for the paternalistic, top-down approach to health education that it took (Farrent and Russell;1985,p14). The demise of the HEC is dealt with in the following chapter, suffice to say here that it trod a careful and, ultimately, unsuccessful path between what it believed the population needed to know, and what the government was prepared to sanction.

The problems with assisting individuals to make informed health choices are well illustrated by general practice. Given that some 75% of people visit their GP every year, it would not be unreasonable to suppose that this would provide a forum for education, or the dissemination of information. As the Royal College of General Practitioners (RCGP) has noted:

> The structure and traditions of British General   Practice are in some ways suited to the development of a style of anticipatory care. (RCGP;1981,p3).

This structure, which places GPs locally and operates the referral system, also has disadvantages. The structure of general practice, according to the Royal College, also acted as a disincentive to longer consultation times because GP's are paid, in part at least, by the size of their patient lists. The incentive under these circumstances was to have larger lists which reduce the amount of consultation time available to each patient. Similarly, it was argued that the use of Primary Health Care Teams could be encouraged by reimbursing a greater proportion of their salaries to GPs. The RCGP report (*Health and Prevention*) highlighted another problem:

> ...we are compelled to write this report largely in ignorance of the extent to which the activities, attitudes and organisation relevant to prevention already exist in general practice in Britain (RCGP;1981a,p8).

The fact that there had been no systematic attempt to utilise the resources a available to general practice was reflected in the lack of information surrounding the extent to which those resources exist. One reason for this was, as Tait observed, that GPs are generally "isolated" in their practice, and therefore deliberate attempts must be made to seek out this sort of information (Tait,*in*, OHE;1985,p24).

The signals both from governments and from General Practice are mixed. The Thatcher governments have shown a marked tendency to favour primary care over and above hospital based services. The Family Practitioner Committees, which had previously only administered General Practice, were strengthened in 1985 by having greater powers to plan and monitor the services provided. This was taken a stage further in 1987 with the publication of *Promoting Better Health* (DHSS). Such initiatives circumvent some of the problems faced by General Practice and which were noted by the Royal College reports. Much depends, however, on the extent to which health promotion and monitoring is successful, particularly given the wide variation in the standards of General Practices that exist. The recent White Paper on the reform of the NHS is a little ambiguous on the question of health promotion (DoH;1989). Within the plans for General Practice it is proposed that GP's should be given the freedom to choose between, for example, using their budgets for out patient facilities, or employing more staff for primary health care teams. Similarly, in 1986 and again in 1989, the present government has proposed to increase the amount of a GP's income that is derived from capitation fees (DHSS;1986, DoH;1989). This, in turn, would presumably act as an incentive to lengthen GP's patient lists. As Allsop has argued, there seems to be some "tensions between practical policy concerns, and ideology." (Allsop, *in*, McCarthy (ed);1989,p66).

It would appear, therefore, that regardless of the fact that "The government is determined that in future much greater emphasis should be given to prevention (DHSS;1977,p3)", in terms of primary prevention at least, this determination has had its limits.

But the problems of this type of approach to prevention are broader than the inability of "governments" to employ the strategy to its full potential. The assumptions upon which this ideology is based are themselves open to question. Central to this philosophy is the contention that: "To a large extent...it is clear that the weight of responsibility for his [her] own state of health lies on the shoulders of the individual him [her] self (DHSS;1976,p38)". However, this is usually found in conjunction with the qualification that: "If the Government is too interventionist it could be regarded as interfering with the liberty of the individual to do as he [she] sees fit with his [her] own life and health (DHSS;1977,p5)". The extent to which governments can suggest or compel certain behaviour in pursuit of health goals is, therefore, problematic. Similarly, and crucially in terms of this study:

> ...it would seem wrong to use resources or interfere
> with individual liberty if there is real doubt whether the
> action proposed will in fact produce the benefits claimed
> for it (DHSS;1977,p6).

This much perhaps is obvious, but the problems that may arise from it do present practical difficulties, for example, when is the doubt real and when is it not; in whose opinion should we trust; what is the level of benefit that we are aiming for? The contentiousness of the scientific evidence relating diet to CHD clearly indicates that suggesting dietary change to consumers, let alone instigating new policies, may rest upon how convinced the government decides to be about the evidence. These questions not only affect the problems of how "interventionist" to be, but also the utility of seeing the individual as being responsible their own health. For example, an extremely cautious approach to the evidence available, coupled with a great concern with the liberty of the individual, could render the notion of individual responsibility for health almost meaningless in the absence of clear health information. There are other corollaries to seeing the individual as being responsible for ill-health. The first, as I mentioned above, is that the cost of prevention is, by definition, reduced. A second is that:

> Implicit in this is the allocation of responsibility, and

blame, for ill-health to the individual and a diffusion of blame and responsibility from government (Allsop; 1984,p178).

This is related both to costs, in that responsibility will not be accepted for those things that the individual should (or should not) be doing for themselves, and to the curative ideology; it is the individuals' fault if they become ill, at which point, the state will repair you. It does not bode well for strong state action to reduce the incidence of CHD if much prevention is seen as necessary because of individual behaviour and administered through that behaviour.

Emphasising the role of the individual places pressure upon the state to create the conditions under which informed decisions can be made. Doyal and Epstein, for example, argue:

> ...the most important problem with this [lifestyle] approach is that the way people live is not simply a matter of individual choice....but is structured in a multitude of ways by their wider social and economic environment (Doyal and Epstein;1983,p16).

On this argument, which I believe to be accurate, simply informing a person that their lifestyle is conducive to ill-health will not be sufficient for them to change that lifestyle. A "consistent" policy in this respect would need to consider the cultural, economic and social circumstances of the individuals concerned, or the broader environmental conditions which may contribute to behaviour patterns (unemployment, divorce, stress, low income, inner cities etc). Only when this can be done, that is, only when a person is fully informed and in a position to affect changes in their lifestyle, can they then be held responsible for not doing so. Even if this is the case, it is still reasonable to argue that the state has responsibilities, for example, with regard to tobacco advertising, providing information, deciding the levels of state benefits etc. Again, returning specifically to CHD, this is important because, insofar as individuals may be held responsible for reducing their risk factors through modifying their lifestyles, they must be in a position to make informed decisions.

This relates to the criticisms of the "lifestyle" approach to health education. The Canterbury Report (1984) on preventing heart disease highlighted the fact that there were a number of different approaches to health education available, but that the most effective was community based; this was also the conclusion of the WHO report (WHO;1982). If lifestyle and behaviour are to some extent at least environmentally determined then it seems reasonable to base health education upon an understanding of communities and community circumstances.

The scope that the available preventive services offer for the reduction of CHD is large, and yet this brief survey has qualified the extent to which they might be used. Too great an emphasis on a life-style approach and the under-utilisation of primary care or health education are quite frequent features of prevention in Britain which may militate against an effective response to CHD.

Heart Disease

As I said in Chapter Three, CHD has been a major cause of death in Britain since before WWII, but there have been a number of factors which have worked against it emerging as a political issue as opposed to a purely medical one.

Throughout the 1920's and the 1930's references can be found to heart disease in the Chief Medical Officer of the Ministry of Health's annual report and the Registrar General's Statistical Survey (Bartley;1985). It becomes clear that there was some confusion at the time as to the "reality" of the rise in the rates of CHD that were being detected. This appears to have centred on two things. Firstly, life expectancy was rising and with it came a rise in the rate of CHD, particularly amongst middle aged men. Secondly, death certification procedures were changing and causes of death which had previously been diagnosed as of the nervous and respiratory system were now more likely to be classified as some sort of heart condition. Bartley (1985,p296) quotes the Registrar General's report for 1926:

> There thus appear to be two causes for the increase since 1911-20 of crude mortality from heart disease....(1) ageing of the population, (2) the rapidly growing tendency to record cardiac degeneration in certifying deaths of old people formerly ascribed simply to such causes as "old age", "bronchitis" etc. [and therefore,] alarmist pronouncements as to increase of mortality from heart disease by the "stress and worry of

126

modern life" may be met with the observation that it is declining (HMSO,1928,pp90-91, *in*, Bartley;1985).

Bartley's argument is that CHD actually rose faster before WWII than afterwards which, to his mind, makes the assumption that it is a disease of affluence questionable. His preferred explanation is that it is, indeed, related to chronic social stress, and not to lifestyles. It is perfectly possible for heart disease to be related to both, given that the major identified risk-factors cannot, in themselves, account for all CHD.

These certification and methodological difficulties were compounded by the fact that the aetiology of the disease was largely unknown. While it was recognised that arteriosclerosis (furring of the arteries) was an important factor, there was still some confusion as to what the causes of it were. Morris (1951) argued that the lack of systematic data on the disease made investigation of its causes very much more difficult but the available evidence seemed to suggest geographical, ethnic and class variations in the disease as well as a possible connection with obesity. He also said that the evidence appeared to support the notion that a "qualitative change" (1951,p70) had taken place during and after WWII: "This, if confirmed, would indicate study of changing modes of life and the changing environment, (Morris;1951,p70)".

At this stage it is not surprising that little was done given that very little was known about the disease. In the Chief Medical Officer's (CMO) report of 1963 (MoH;1964) concrete policy proposals were forwarded and it was recognised that fats in the diet may contribute to CHD. The CMO referred to research that had emanated from the United States which implicated soft drinking water and diet although he stressed that: "The role of saturated and unsaturated fat.....are still in the investigative stage (MoH;1964,p182)."

Hospital-centred Coronary Care Units had already been established unilaterally by health professionals. The logic behind these units was that deaths from heart failure usually came within two hours of a victim having an attack, and before they could receive medical treatment. Early treatment could save lives. The 1963 report endorsed the extension of these units to mobile centres and asked for their progress to be monitored. McLachlan (1973) has argued that, in fact, these units were not particularly successful. Given the scale of the problem, they could never have offered a solution, but it is interesting to note that these innovations were generated within the structure of the NHS and were, in the first instance at least, a curative, treatment based response. The CMO had recognised the limitations of such an approach:

If some form of easily applied and well-tolerated preventive treatment were available it might be satisfactory to recommend this for all persons falling within the high risk group (MoH;1964,p182).

This is interesting because of the assumptions that it rests upon. Prevention would have to be "administered" in a clinical fashion and it would apply to the "high risk group" alone. Neither of these are particularly surprising except that they became persistent features of the official line on heart disease.

For the rest of the 1960's there appears to be very little that was said on what should be done about heart disease. This changed in 1970 with the appointment of a COMA panel to consider the topic of *Diet and Heart Disease.*(DHSS;1974). The panel took four years to survey the literature available and the report was published in 1974. Publication of the report does not appear to have had any significant political impact. It was not unanimous, and this would have detracted from its authoritativeness, but there was little public discussion of its contents at all, save in medical journals. The recommendations of the report were:

1. There should be a reduction in the consumption of saturated fat.
2. This should *not* be compensated for by an increase in Polyunsaturated Fatty Acids (PUFA's).
3. Sugar consumption should remain the same.
4. Salt consumption should remain the same (DHSS;1974).

The COMA report did not, therefore, become the basis of what might be called a "policy" as no new initiatives were taken to adopt or promote the recommendations. Lord Ennals, the then Secretary of State for the Social Services, appears to blame the "experts":

When I was Secretary of State for the Social Services from 1976 to 1979 it was frankly impossible to get an agreed conclusion from the panel (Ennals;1984,p381).
I couldn't get the medics, the nutritionists, the food scientists to agree on anything. I now realise that half the experts on my advisory committees were paid by one side of the food industry or another. (Ennals;1986, *quoted in,* Cannon;1987,p299).

These are two different explanations (or justifications) for the same political outcome. The controversy rested not only on the nature of the evidence itself, but also on the responsibilities that were incumbent upon professionals when giving advice to the general public. The political context of the report had not escaped the notice of professionals:

> The implications of the panels recommendations for the food industry, for government food regulations and subsidies and even for the EEC agricultural arrangements will need to be carefully studied (BMJ;1974,).

Whether Ennals' contention that these experts were employed by the food industry can explain their differences of opinion is more difficult to establish. Cannon (1987) is of the opinion that the links between industry and science are implicated in scientific reports which reflect a particular commercial ideology. Similarly, it is known that the food industry did its best to "sink" the COMA recommendations when they arrived in MAFF (Personal Correspondence (O); 1986). Again, such a move would be consistent with industry disliking constraints on its competitiveness.

This is also borne out by the DHSS's reaction to the Public Expenditure Committee's Sub-Committee recommendations that:

> Information about fats should be placed before the public in order to show up clearly the risks from a high intake of saturated fats, to encourage people to moderate their fat intake or switch to polyunsaturated fats.
> The proportion of saturated fat and polyunsaturated fats should appear on the labels of manufactured foods. DHSS (DHSS;1977,p79-80).

The first of these recommendations was accepted with reservations, and the second was put under consideration. In fact, it was not until the publication of another COMA report in 1984 that these "considerations" were acted upon, and even now these labels are not enforceable until they gain EC approval. The response of the DHSS to recommendations which might affect commercial interests were reasonably consistent and the above examples are typical.

Throughout the 1970's and the early 1980's, commercial constraints and divided professional opinion placed the DHSS in a difficult position. On the one hand, it has accepted the likelihood of the relationship between diet and heart disease, while on the other hand, it has been extremely reluctant to do anything about it (DHSS;1976(a),p62. 1977,p41, 1979,p71-72, 1981,p44).

The DHSS's reluctance to provide strong dietary guidelines affected its relationship with the Health Education Council (HEC). Farrant and Russell (1985) document the production the *Beating Heart Disease* publicity booklet, arguing that after the publication of the booklet *Prevention and Health:Avoiding Heart Attacks* (DHSS;1981 as above) the DHSS pressured the HEC to extend its programme on heart disease prevention:

> However, just as Beating Heart Disease was about to go to print, it was made clear to the HEC that the DHSS did not accept the quantified dietary goals quoted in the draft HEC Programme. It was made clear that the DHSS would object in the strongest possible terms to the publication of the objectives in their current quantified form, especially since a committee (COMA) was being set up ..on this very subject. Reference was also made to the possibly adverse reaction of the Food Manufacturers Foundation [they meant Federation] to such advice being published (Farrant and Russell;1985,43).

Once again there is the connection between the actions of the DHSS and the commercial repercussions of those actions. The DHSS consistently refused to indicate the *level* of reduction in saturated fat that it thought would be prudent, and it extended this refusal to the HEC as well.

In 1976, the Royal College of Physicians and the Cardiac Society published a report named *Prevention of Coronary Heart Disease* in which it did quantify the levels of fat that it thought would be reasonable (towards 35% of total calories; 1976,p230). But the report was equally interesting because it was the first British source to argue that CHD was an essentially preventable disease. The response of the DHSS was to ask the COMA panel to reconsider their 1974 recommendations, and the panel duly came to the same conclusions as before.

The "story" of diet and heart disease as an emerging political issue is largely one of contending interpretations of the actions and motives of governments - this will remain the case in the following chapter. Initially, the curative response of health professionals was predictable given the resources at their disposal, the scale of the problem, and the level of knowledge concerning the risk-factors involved.

After the publication of the 1974 COMA report, however, it appears that even though reductions in the level of saturated fat consumption were recommended, the DHSS was extremely reluctant to emphasise this particular risk-factor. It seems there was almost certainly a strong economic/commercial reasoning behind this reluctance. As Sir Donald Acheson, the present Chief Medical Officer of the Department of Health, has observed:

> It is a ...difficult matter for it [the government] to propose that the consumption of pleasurable but perhaps harmful [food] factors should be reduced, particularly when the employment and prosperity of a large part of the nation depend on the production of these substances (Acheson;1986,p137).

The combination of these difficulties and the medical profession's inability to produce a British consensus before the 1980's, produced a political vacuum. The steadily emerging body of knowledge relating diet to many diseases, not just heart disease, required a political lead and/or strong opinions from the state which was not forthcoming. I will argue in the following chapter that it is for this reason that the state was eventually forced to take the problem of diet and heart disease more seriously.

Conclusion

We saw in the last chapter that despite the existence of a post-WWII nutrition policy, that policy did not seem particularly well suited to tackling the problems of dietary change in Britain.

In this chapter, we have explored features of the health care system which may also help to promote that change. Certain conclusions seem to suggest themselves. The power of professionals is firmly rooted in the health care system and so we can anticipate that where this system can be utilised for dietary change, it will be. However, we also know that lifestyle and commercial changes will need to be made, and it is by no means clear that professionals are in a position to promote changes of this sort.

We also know that the lifestyle approach is often favoured by governments because it is cheap and it places the burden of responsibility upon the individual. However, for such a scheme to work, consumers have to be extremely well informed and be in a position to comply with the information they are given. This too is often problematic particularly if the DOH has shown a marked reluctance in the past to quantify how much dietary change consumers should be aiming for.

Finally, we can conclude that preventive services are well placed to reduce the incidence of CHD but historically have been used in "at-risk" (vulnerable) strategies, and not for population level prevention. In all these cases, the scope for action on the part of the health care system has been constrained in the past by (1) a concern for the freedom of individuals to choose lifestyles, and (2) the possible economic consequences of state intervention on the demand side of food.

7 The COMA Report

In 1984, the DHSS accepted a report on *Diet and Cardiovascular Disease* from its advisory body, the Committee on the Medical Aspects of Food Policy (COMA). The recommendations of the report have formed the basis for the government's strategy to reduce CHD largely, although not exclusively, through dietary change.

We already know that any policies of this sort are going to involve what is now the Department of Health (DoH) and the Ministry of Agriculture Fisheries and Food (MAFF) in, as yet, unquantified proportions. So, the COMA report gives us the opportunity to test some of the more obvious hypothesis we have made about the nature of food and health policies in Britain. Does MAFF continue to exert a strong degree of control over food-related policies and is this control compatible with genuine dietary change? Will professionals have the resources to force through dietary changes if necessary? How will the DoH respond to recommendations which suggest its role should involve greater advocacy for dietary change?

In the preceding chapters I have argued that in all these instances there is little historical precedent for such recommendations to be fully implemented. Dietary change has to overcome some serious ideological, institutional and economic hurdles to be successful and would require "heroic" policies.

This chapter begins with an account of another report (NACNE) which preceded COMA, and which was the primary reason why the government commissioned COMA to consider diet and cardiovascular disease. This is followed by the recommendations of the COMA report itself and the response of the government to those recommendations. The chapter ends with a discussion and evaluation of government policies.

The NACNE Report

The story of the NACNE report is important in three respects. Firstly, it confirms many of the themes that I tried to develop in the previous chapter, for example, the link between industry and health policies. Secondly, it was because of the existence of this report that the DHSS commissioned *Diet and Cardiovascular Disease* (DHSS:1984) which was to become the blueprint for policy on the prevention of heart disease. Thirdly, the NACNE report was to act as a catalyst for many local food policies and partially filled the "guideline" vacuum left by the DHSS. The controversial circumstances surrounding the publication of the NACNE report politicised dietary change and placed the issue on the political agenda.

Throughout the post-war period conventional views on what constituted a "healthful" diet, were gradually changing. While this did not bring any major political response from any government, it did not go entirely unnoticed. In 1973 the Secretary of State at the DHSS (Sir Keith Joseph) initiated a working party of DHSS officials, the Health Education Council (HEC) and the British Nutrition Foundation[1] (BNF). This group was supposed to advise the DHSS on the changes in nutritional orthodoxy, and to suggest ways in which this might be incorporated into nutrition education (Walker and Cannon;1985).

It was not until 1979, however, that the National Advisory Committee on Nutrition Education (NACNE) was established and began to tackle the task of deciding what constituted the new nutritional orthodoxy. It was decided

---

[1] The British Nutrition Foundation is an industry-funded research organisation.

that a sub-committee should be set up to make a comprehensive survey of the available evidence, and having done so, report to the main committee. This report, became known as the NACNE report. The membership of the committee included representatives from: "...the practitioners of nutrition education, the food industry, DHSS and MAFF, BNF, HEC and the Scottish Health Education Group, and the academic community (HEC;1983,p7)".

The report went through three drafts, none of which were acceptable to MAFF or the then DHSS. This appears to be because the sub-committee exceeded its terms of reference by formulating dietary guidelines rather than simply stating the new orthodoxy. After the third draft was finished, in April 1983, the existence of the report became public knowledge. A copy was leaked to the Sunday Times and a front page article appeared (Sunday Times;1983,p1). From this point on, the debate surrounding dietary change became much more political because it was argued in the Sunday Times article that the governments' actions amounted to suppression.

The NACNE report was politically significant for a number of reasons, not least because it was published by the HEC and so was an authoritative and respectable source of information. It covered most of the contentious nutritional issues which had been avoided by the DHSS and recommended the following:

Table 7.0.

Salt.	Should be reduced by 50%
Sugar.	Should be reduced by 50%
Fibre.	Should be increased by 50%
Fats.	Should be reduced by 25%, saturated fats by 50%.
Alcohol.	Should be reduced by 33%.

Source: HEC;1983.

Not only was the NACNE report confident in the recommendations it made, it quantified them as well.

The response of local authorities, schools and health authorities to the report demonstrates that these agencies had wanted guidance from the centre. A report published by the Bradford Food Policy Research Group notes that after the publication of the NACNE report there was a large increase in the number of local food policies (Montague;1985) and goes on to distinguish between policies adopted before and after the publication of the NACNE report, implying that its publication was something of a landmark. The importance of the report appears to be that it suggested what a "healthful" diet might be, and quantified the changes. It was then possible for local authorities, for example, to apply nutritional standards to the food they served to their staff and clients.

Unsurprisingly, the government distanced itself from the report. Two members of the full NACNE committee have said independently that the reason the COMA panel was convened at that particular time (1981) was so that it could narrow the terms of the dietary change debate and delay comment or action on the NACNE report (Personal Correspondence (A) and (D); 1987 and 1986):

> Instituting the COMA Report at a time when the NACNE report seemed highly controversial, was a mechanism whereby the Government could properly dissociate itself from any new policy statement, whilst currently reconsidering their own (James, *in*, Royal Society; 1989,p1).

In a written reply to a question from J. Michael Shersby MP (a director of the Sugar Bureau) a Junior Health Minister confirmed that the NACNE report was not an official document and did not represent government policy (Patten;1984,p194-195). Indeed, Shersby denied that the report existed, arguing that it was simply the findings of an ad hoc working group (Personal Correspondence (E);1986). This is a position adopted by much of industry.

While it is impossible to know the precise reasons why the government were unwilling to accommodate the recommendations of the NACNE report its position is consistent with the response to the 1974 COMA report and to preventive medicine in general. The commercial effects of the recommendations outlined above would have touched on farming and food manufacturing industries, in some cases aiming to reduce consumption by between one third and a half. Similarly, the quantification of change implies extending responsibilities beyond simply advising the general public and toward actively achieving targets.

By accepting new targets across a range of food areas there is an implicit shift away from merely regulating the supply side of the food market toward the manipulation of demand. This is something that has little historical precedent and tends to conflict with principle of individual freedom of choice. It also interferes with the free operation of the market, because the guidelines would favour some products over and above others.

Until the DHSS and MAFF became aware of the NACNE report, official or quasi-official guidelines on the emerging nutritional orthodoxy were vague and/or incomplete. After publication the issue could no longer be controlled; it had entered the political agenda and required a positive political response. The response of the government was the acceptance and publication of the 1984 COMA report on *Diet and Cardiovascular Disease*.

The COMA Report

The government commissioned the 1984 COMA report by default rather than by design. Unlike information from other sources, there are certain procedural peculiarities which make COMA a favoured source.

The terms of reference of COMA panels can be chosen by the DoH although COMA can suggest areas it thinks are worth looking at. The membership of the panel is chosen by the DoH. Again, this may or may not be important, but there is evidence to suggest that this procedural control can be manipulated. For example, the membership of the 1984 panel have been said to represent a more "conservative" sample of the experts available to the DHSS (Personal Correspondence (D);1986).

While the reports represent the considered opinions of the elite professionals on the panel, they are written by civil servants, and then approved by the panel afterwards. I will expand on this point later. Finally, it is possible for the timing of the reports to be politically controlled.

These are the more obvious differences between the COMA report and, for example, the NACNE report of 1983, the Royal College report of 1976, or the BMA report of 1986. There are other, more intangible differences which may also be important:

> One of the great benefits of the COMA Panel Report in my view was that it had been organized by the Government, and Panellists felt under considerable pressure to produce a report which would be accepted by Government (James, *in*, Royal Society;1989,p2).

So, without questioning the integrity of the COMA panel itself, there appear both tangible and intangible pressures under which the report was written.

The COMA report was published in 1984 and accepted by the government immediately.

The recommendations of the report were directed at 5 distinct sectors of the community; the general public; medical practitioners; those working in the food chain; professionals and the Government.

The recommendations to the general public included such things as reducing total fat consumption to 35% of calories, and saturated fat to no more than 15%; not increasing intakes of sugar or salt; avoiding obesity, excessive alcohol and smoking; and increasing consumption of fibre.

Medical practitioners were urged to identify those "at risk" and give vigorous dietary advice to those patients.

COMA wanted the food industry to give more information on food labels and to make that information easy to understand particularly on butter, margarine, cooking fats and edible oils and "all other foods with a fat content of more than 10% by weight, or which are major contributors to fat intake". There were recommendations to label alcoholic beverages of more than 1.2% alcohol by volume and to make low fat and low salt products available.

An appeal was made to the DoH, the Royal College of Physicians of London (RCPL) and the British Cardiac Society to establish joint machinery for an on going review of CHD. The recommendations to government were:

(1) The general population should be educated into good eating habits and the value of physical activity; this process should begin in schools.

(2) There should be consultations with the food industry to improve public knowledge of the composition of foods and public awareness of the alcohol content of alcoholic drinks. This should lead, ultimately, to the availability of low fat and low salt products, legislation and codes of practice.

(3) Consideration should be given to ways and means of encouraging the production of leaner carcasses in sheep, cattle and pigs (for example by adjustments to the carcass grading systems).

(4) Consideration should be given to ways and means of removing from the Common Agricultural Policy those elements which discourage individuals and families from implementing recommendations for dietary change.

(5) A cost/benefit enquiry should be made on identifying those more at risk of CHD. There should also be encouragement given to research which can find a cheaper way of measuring blood lipids and blood pressure.

The way that responsibilities have been divided up between the five groups is interesting. The recommendation to reduce overall fat consumption by a

138

quarter is directed at the general public, and not at the government. So, even though there are now quantified targets the government is not responsible for achieving them. Again, the individual is seen as the person primarily responsible for avoiding the circumstances and conditions which contribute to their ill-health.

The recommendations to the food industry impinge on many of the traditional responsibilities of MAFF. These are mostly concerned with food and drink labelling, and suggest industry is expected to respond to the panel's recommendations, independently of any joint initiatives that it may take with MAFF. While fat labelling was seen as the responsibility of government, labelling on sugar and salt (both of which are indirectly related to CHD) was left to the food industry itself.

Each sector of the community is considered independently from the other, and the report does not relate the responsibilities they have attributed to them back to their financial or political source (ie. government). In other words, dealing with these sectors separately tends to disperse responsibilities which in reality would need the active support of central government. Whether the recommendations are directed at the government or not most, if not all, will be mediated through it.

Finally, of the five recommendations, three were the responsibility of MAFF, one fell to the DHSS and the other to both the DHSS and the Department of Education and Science (DES). The willingness and ability of MAFF to accommodate professional opinion on dietary change is, therefore, crucial.

Implementing COMA

In a sparsely attended Commons debate in 1984, John Patten, a junior Health Minister, gave the government's response to the publication of the COMA report (Hansard;1984,p147-154). It was "welcomed" and although no firm commitments could be made at that stage "consultations" between government and interested parties would take place. The initiator of the debate, Jonathon Aiken, stressed the importance that should be attached to education and food labelling. This theme was also pursued in a House of Lords debate on the report when the government spokes-person argued strongly in favour of education and information (Earl of Caithness;1984,p388) .

A MAFF press release of 1985 sets out in more detail the policies of both MAFF and the DHSS. There are proposals on fat labelling, alcoholic drinks, carcass grading, blood lipid detection, health education and the CAP. The notice says: "We are ......working towards implementing all the COMA recommendations to Government (MAFF;1985,p1)".

While some recommendations have been fully accepted others have not. From the 1977 DHSS report (*Prevention and Health*) is was clear that the funding of research was something that the DHSS was willing to undertake and this has happened with blood lipids and blood pressure. Similarly, the DHSS set up a new Unit on Coronary Heart Disease within its own department and has sponsored research into how publicity campaigns might be received by consumers.

These "in-house" initiatives appear to be easily accommodated by the DoH, it is only when they deal more directly with the public that their actions become more constrained.

Food Labelling In 1984, MAFF, in conjunction with the Consumers Association and the National Consumer Council, commissioned a study of "Consumer Attitudes to and Understanding of Nutrition Labelling" (BMRB;1985 and Susie Fisher;1985). The object of the exercise was:

> ...to obtain information on the attitudes to nutrition labelling, and to assess the most appropriate ways of presenting the information such that it is easily understood and useful to the consumer (BMRB;1985,p1).

The report found that consumers were confused over certain words such as kilo-joules, carbohydrates, fatty acids, RDA (Recommended Daily Amount/Allowance), energy, sodium, per serving/per 100g. They preferred plain English; disliked colour-coding; preferred charts but used numerical presentations more effectively. Highly detailed tables were not liked.

Following the research, MAFF issued its discussion paper on the proposals for both the *Fat Content of Food (Labelling) Regulations* and its guidelines on *Nutrition Labelling* (MAFF;1986(a), MAFF;1986(b)).

The basic format for fat content labelling was that all foods would be labelled with their actual fat content plus the level of "saturates"; food sold "loose" would have to have a notice showing its fat content; milk bottle lids would show the level of fat (by colour of the lid); the term "typical value" would be applied to the labels, etc.

The provisional guidelines for nutrition labelling were a little more complicated because they required food labels to have a specified format. Altogether there were three groups of information that were proposed for food labels. Group A included fat, protein, carbohydrate and energy. The fat must be broken down into fat and saturates, as the *Fat Content Labelling Regulations* required. The manufacturers could, if they wanted, label for energy as well but if they did, they must also label for protein and carbohydrate . In Group B sodium (salt) could be declared and the carbohydrates broken down to show sugars separately. This could only be done if all of the Group A nutrients were listed first. The same applied for nutrients in Group C. Again, once Groups A and B had been labelled then Group C (vitamins and minerals) could also be included. All these formats had been discussed with industry before they were circulated.

The general format of the nutrition labels is almost identical with the FAO/WHO Codex Alimentarius system that will be adopted by the EEC in 1992. At the moment, food labels are covered by Council Directive (79/112) of 1978 which says things like the name of the product, a list of ingredients, a date of minimum durability, specific storage conditions and the like " alone shall be compulsory on the labelling of foodstuffs" (European Commission;1979,p33/3). Article 15 allows further details only if it is for the "protection of public health". MAFF reluctantly decided to invoke Article 15 so that they could require fat content labelling (Personal Correspondence (F);1986) but were not prepared to do it for any other purpose. Even so, the decision on fat labelling would have to be agreed by the Commission, and is still being considered. It was pointed out by the National Forum report however:

> MAFF blames the delay in the introduction even of mandatory fat labelling on opposition from the EEC. It fears that a British initiative in this area.....will contravene the EEC directive on food labelling. This view has been challenged on the basis of lack of precedent (National Forum;1988,p107).

The new system will not be compulsory for member states because it is a "Recommendation of the Commission" which is not binding. The question arises whether devising a new labelling system was indeed part of MAFF's response to the COMA report, or simply part of Britain's preparation for the Single European Act.

Even though industry had been partly responsible for framing the draft proposals, the reaction of the meat and dairy sectors in particular was not entirely favourable. The Dairy Trade Federation argued that simply making fat content labelling compulsory was putting the industry at a competitive disadvantage. Under this system the industry would not necessarily be able to advertise the fact that their products are high in protein or calcium, while those who produced low fat products of dubious nutritional value, would be given a competitive advantage (Personal Correspondence (G);1986). The NFU were similarly unimpressed by compulsory fat content labelling:

> In principle, the proposal to label only the fat content of
> food is not acceptable as it will single out one
> constituent of the food stuff and will thus suggest that
> fat is a particular danger to health (Dalzell;1985,p1).

The NFU were also unconvinced that it was possible to accurately specify the fat content of meat, particularly with products which were not made to uniform specifications eg. cuts of meat.

The Bacon and Meat Manufacturers Association (BMMA) were upset by the Meat Traders Association's attempt to get an exemption from the fat content regulations. It was opposed by the BMMA, again, on the grounds that this would give butchers an advantage over other meat manufacturers (Personal Correspondence (H);1987).

In all three examples, therefore, we see perhaps what might be expected given the characterisation of the food industry presented in Chapter Four. Industry wants to know how the proposals from MAFF are going to affect its competitiveness.

The criticisms of consumer groups have, not surprisingly, been of a different nature. While industry was preoccupied with the fat content labelling regulations, consumer groups criticised the nutritional labelling regulations. The Consumers Association, for example, noted that the voluntary guidelines did not demand the inclusion of fibre, sugar and salt (Consumers Association;1986). The National Consumer Council criticised, amongst other things, the fact that there were five possible formats for nutrition labels, and suggested that two would be ample (NCC;1986). The London Food Commission generally welcomed the proposals on fat content labelling but reserved judgement on the implementation period (2 years after presentation to Parliament), the basis for calculation (ie. wet or dry weight), exempting milk from labelling and the use of typical values without adequate policing methods (Luba and Cole-Hamilton;1986).

There were also objections about the terminology that was to be used on the labels, particularly where it ran contrary to the research findings on what was best understood by consumers. Even under the voluntary guidelines the term carbohydrate (which includes both sugars and starches) does not have to be broken down to show whether it refers to sugars or starches unless the manufacturer wishes to label from Group B. A consumer would not necessarily know whether a product which was high in "carbohydrates" was a high sugar or a high starch product - it may be neither, or it may be both. It was also proposed that the term "sodium" should be used instead of salt, despite the research showing that 69% of respondents thought people should cut down on salt, and 41% thought intake of sodium should stay the same. Equally, the research indicated a great deal of confusion among consumers over the differences between, and meanings of, calories, energy, kilo calories and kilo joules which either measure or describe the same thing. "Calories" were generally well known, but the draft guidelines proposed expressing energy in terms of kilo joules and kilo calories which were not generally understood.

When the final regulations were announced in 1987, there were very few changes to the draft guidelines. The fat regulations were to remain broadly the same, the only major change being that it would no longer be necessary to declare total fat as well as saturated fat content-only saturated fat content was required. Nutritional labels were left very much the same except that now only four formats are possible whereas before there were five. The nutritional labelling is still only voluntary.

From the evidence available, it appears that industry has done particularly well out of these proposals. The nutrition labelling guidelines have given all sectors broadly what they wanted, that is, the opportunity to present information which is favourable to their products. For example, breakfast cereal, which is often fortified, will display the full labelling format which includes vitamins and minerals in the final Group. On the other hand, a product such as chocolate (which is high in sugar) will only display Group A, which means it does not have to declare the sugar content. This supports a point made earlier, that the bottom line for industry is that it must remain innovative and competitive. There is no meaningful sense in which the industry itself can be relied upon to be self-regulating when these principles are challenged.

The amendment to fat content labelling means that products which are high in Trans Fatty Acids (thought to have a similar physiological effect to saturated fat) will not have to contain a full declaration of fats and it also means that consumers are unaware of the ratio of saturated to polyunsaturated fat in a product.

The MAFF press release of 1985 implies that full nutritional labelling was not originally considered by MAFF:

> Representatives of the food industry have asked the government to consider full nutrition labelling of all foods covering such things as energy, protein and carbohydrate content as well as fat content (MAFF;1985,p2).

Why did the food industry ask MAFF to do this? The only plausible explanation is that full nutrition labelling not only allows manufacturers to be selective in the information that they give to consumers, it also acts to divert attention away from the fat content.

This apparent compliance with the wishes of the food industry runs in direct contradiction to the research into consumer attitudes to food labels, the recommendations of the COMA report, and indeed, the principle that the state can aid preventive medicine through providing consumers with useful information. Thus, not only does the policy on food labelling fail to fulfil the minimal commitment to effective prevention that has historically been accepted by British governments, it also falls short of the expressed intentions of the government (in both Houses of Parliament) to have consumer-led changes in dietary habits.

Health Education The COMA recommendations on health education, diet and cardiovascular disease were aimed at health educators and the government. To the health educators "....advice should be given on how to construct diets and regulate physical activity.." (DHSS;1984,p9). To government, COMA recommended that "....means should be found to educate the general population ....in habits of eating and physical activity...." and that this process should begin schools (DHSS;1984,p11).

Until recently (April 1987), health education at a national level was the responsibility of the Health Education Council (HEC). The HEC was a Quango funded by the DHSS and was abolished to reconvene as a Special Health Authority under the DHSS. This was the culmination of a succession of disagreements and confrontations between the HEC and DHSS. The example of the pamphlet *Beating Heart Disease* which was effectively edited by the DHSS was given in an earlier chapter. Of course, the HEC also published the NACNE report, although were subsequently prevented by the DHSS from quoting it as an authoritative source. This, in itself, must have created tensions between the two.

One outcome of the COMA recommendation to government was the production of *Eating for a Healthier Heart*, a leaflet from the British Nutrition Foundation (BNF) and the HEC. These two bodies now made up the newly formed Joint Advisory Committee on Nutrition Education (JACNE) as by now NACNE had been abolished.

The story of the JACNE leaflet bears a great deal of resemblance to that of the NACNE report. There were DHSS and MAFF observers on the committee and the first draft was returned by the DHSS saying that the "Government" was not happy with it. Some suggestions were given as to changes that might be made and those which were of a technical nature were largely included. For example, a proposal for consumers to substitute vegeburgers for beefburgers was dropped after it was discovered they contained the same amount of fat (Personal Correspondence (B);1987).

The tension between JACNE and the DHSS did not reside in the technical issues but rather in the structure of the leaflet and the scope of its information. It was clear to the committee that the government (MAFF and the DHSS) were having trouble reconciling the information in the leaflet with the problems it would cause the dairy industry (Personal Correspondence (A);1987). In other words, telling consumers that dairy products might cause CHD might be expected to have commercial repercussion. The issue was only resolved when the Chairperson of JACNE threatened to resign and the letter he had sent the DHSS was leaked to the Sunday Times (Gillie;1985). The following Monday an article appeared in The Guardian (Veitch;1985), and on the Tuesday the DHSS gave the go-ahead for the leaflet to be printed. Shortly afterwards JACNE was abolished.

The JACNE leaflet, on first appraisal at least, meets the requirements of the COMA recommendations on reducing the consumption of fats and saturated fats. But, the COMA recommendations on sugar, salt and alcohol have been omitted. It has also been argued that the questionnaire format and the over-simplistic approach of the leaflet, are actually unhelpful to consumers. A health education official has said that this was the only publication that had ever been returned to the HEC because of its inaffectiveness (Personal Correspondence (A);1987).

The HEC decided to stop printing the JACNE leaflet, and to replace it with its own *Guide to Healthy Eating* (HEC;1986). In contrast to *Eating for a Healthier Heart*, this covered a range of foods and drinks, and contained strong recommendations to the general public, on, for example, misleading food descriptions. It also suggested that consumers should campaign for changes in the food they eat by writing to food manufacturers or MAFF! (HEC;1986,p25).

The government distanced itself from the NACNE report because its scope was unacceptable, and the same reasoning applies to the JACNE leaflet. The government wished to confine the issue of dietary change to the specific issue of CHD. The HEC leaflet again broadened the scope of the issue and even attempted to further politicise the area by encouraging consumers to comment on the food supply.

The concern of the government, therefore, was not so much to implement the COMA recommendations as to limit dietary change as a political issue. This is entirely understandable because we know from Chapters Four, Five and Six that the government has found itself in an unusual position. Historically, there has been little need to re-define consumption patterns, or to damage parts of the food industry by advising consumers not to eat certain products. Perhaps we should not be surprised that the strategy adopted favours the most entrenched interests at the expense of consumers. Nevertheless, if this conceptualisation is correct, then it does qualify how successful a consumer-led, lifestyle approach to dietary change can be.

Another response of the government to the COMA recommendations has been a publicity campaign, the Look After Your Heart campaign (LAYH), which has now become a programme. This followed the high profile approaches originally used in the Heroin and AIDS campaigns and is run by the new Health Education Authority (HEA).

It was announced in the House of Lords in late 1986 that the campaign would have a budget of £1-2m initially - this has now risen to £5m. The first phase, to last 12-18 months, was to raise awareness and would take a multifactoral approach, that is, it would emphasise all the risk factors associated with CHD, not only diet. Initially, the campaign's approach was to focus on the workplace and then spread out into the community (BSSRS;1986). It targets the largest employers (large companies and local authorities, for example) and promotes anti-coronary policies within the workplace. In essence, the HEA use the programme as an "umbrella " to coordinate the work of employers, local authorities, health authorities, voluntary organisations etc (Personal Correspondence (J);1988). The Authority is not in a position, financially, to take the full burden health education and so takes the best strategy available to it - its projected budget for 1990-95 is approximately £29m p.a. These resource problems were noticed in a National Audit Office (NAO) report, although under-funding was not mentioned explicitly:

> ...the NAO noted that the campaign strategy lacks
> quantified targets and estimates of the resources and
> funding necessary to meet its objectives (NAO;1989,
> p13).

Of course, the absence of quantified targets is nothing new although the HEA has now accepted the World Health Organisation's target of reducing CHD amongst the under 65's by 15% by the year 2000.

Although the HEA advertised it as the "biggest anti-coronary policy in the world", the programme is under-funded and has to compete with the advertising budgets of food companies and the tobacco industry which amount to nearly £1b p.a. (Walker and Cannon;1985, p62 and Cannon;187,p 73). Despite the target of a 15% reduction in CHD, it is likely that the fall in CHD would have continued anyway because of changes in smoking and exercise habits, particularly amongst the middle classes. The difficulty for any policy designed to reduce the incidence of CHD, or indeed to promote dietary change in general, is to reach those parts of the population who would not otherwise have changed their lifestyles:

> Experience gained in trials designed to   test   the
> effect   of   risk   factor   intervention   on   the
> incidence   of   coronary   heart   disease   has   shown
> repeatedly that compliance depends critically upon
> the level and quality of   counselling to participants.
> (DHSS;1984, p9).

This type of counselling is not undertaken by the HEA, rather, it is the job of the HEA to encourage health authorities to promote this work within primary health care teams (PHCT's). It hopes to have 30% more PHCT's doing this type of work by 1993 (HEA;1989). In all these initiatives, success will depend not only on the strategy adopted but also on the resources that are available. There have been no extra resources made available to health authorities to prevent CHD and so it must be assumed that the success of the LAHY programme will, in large part, depend on the persuasiveness of the HEA.

Schools The recommendation to begin education in schools was part of a wider one which deals with education of the general population. The wording of the recommendation leaves the "means" of achieving such education to the discretion of the government.

The official response of the government has been to amend the Home Economics Syllabus to incorporate the findings of the COMA panel. While this is laudable in itself it has to be seen in context, because there are many factors affecting schools which have not been dealt with.

Nutritional standards for school meals were abolished by the 1980 Education Act and this relieved local authorities of responsibility for providing meals which conformed to certain nutritional standards. Consequently, one of the main planks of a policy for dietary change was lost for reasons other than nutrition. Similarly, EEC subsidies on school milk are now only available for whole and semi-skimmed milk, and not for skimmed milk as they were in the past (European Commission;1985).

The onus is, therefore, on the LEA's to accommodate dietary advice within the existing budgets and at their own discretion. Central government has now revised guidelines to them (as well as "hospitals ...and many catering establishments") but these are only guidelines, and they have to be accommodated within existing budgets:

> With the competition for use of local education authority resources there is real concern that national emphasis on nutritional standards is insufficient for the issue to be given priority locally (National Forum;1988,p.109).
> In the summer of 1987 the Government announced its plans to reform the education system and published proposals for a national curriculum. Health education and home economics were not proposed as core or foundation subjects....(National Forum;1988,p109).

At the time of the de-regulation of school meals, Mrs. Thatcher conceded that the quality of meals in schools and the food normally eaten during school hours would be kept under surveillance by the government. This was done by a COMA panel and the results published in a report *The Diets of British Schoolchildren* (Wenlock et al;1986, Veitch;1986). The fate of this report was similar to that of the NACNE report and the JACNE leaflet (Fletcher;1986). The publication of the report had been delayed by the DoH without explanation. When it was published, the standards of schoolchildren's diets bore little resemblance to the COMA recommendations. For example, children were generally worse fed at

148

school than they were at home and they ate too much salt, sugar and fat, and too little fibre. Sadly, the government had committed itself to two separate policy goals which are almost entirely contradictory. On the one hand there was strict control of public expenditure and the withdrawal of the state on nutritional standards, while on the other hand, there is a stated commitment to beginning a process of education on diet and CHD in schools.

There are other opportunities which also seem to have been missed. Changing the General Education syllabus to include diet (about half of pupils have this type of course in their schools); the re-introduction of nutritional standards in school meals; a greater share of the National Curriculum to physical education (only 5% of the timetable is proposed for this at the moment); and stricter controls over the publicity material from industry that can be distributed in schools. An example of this type of material was a video made for schools by the National Dairy Council, which subsequently figured on BBC TV (O'Donnel Investigates). The video contained comparisons which gave the impression that dairy products (ice cream) were no higher in fat than fruit.

Another example comes from the Meat and Livestock Commission. In an attempt to launch a counter-offensive against the health lobby (and vegetarianism in particular), schools are seen as places in which the industry can get across a positive picture of meat:

> The industry can act to minimise the affects [of adverse
> publicity] by:
> intensifying the educational programmes in schools and
> elsewhere (Harrington;1985,p24).

Schools clearly do offer opportunities for the state to affect the future lifestyles of young people. The policy as it stands, however, gives no clear indication of how successful such a strategy can be if it does not take all, or even most, of the opportunities available. Again, we return to the point that there will be effects from this policy, but they are likely to be arbitrary and haphazard.

Encouraging Leaner Carcasses There are many ways of reducing the amount of saturated fat in the food chain. Some can be implemented almost immediately (changes in milk quotas for example); others could take many years (selective breeding). The Common Agricultural Policy (CAP) will be dealt with in a later section, at the moment we will look specifically at the COMA recommendation to produce leaner meat.

Producing fatter animals is far more expensive than producing leaner ones. It takes 5kg of feed to produce 1kg of fat and if fat production was reduced by 17% per annum, it would save 2.4m tonnes of animal feed with a value of £200,000,000 pounds. In the final stages, 65% of cattle's weight gain is pure fat. Slaughtering animals earlier would, therefore, reduce the amount of feed they needed and increase the ratio of lean meat in the carcass. (Jones;1986,p13).

The UK livestock industry produces about 945,000 tonnes of fat per annum:

Table 7.1. Production of fat in British livestock industry in tonnes.

Cattle	450,000.
Sheep	80,000.
Pigs	400,000.

Source: Jones;Undated, p4-7.

If the COMA recommendations were implemented (ie. reducing saturated fat by 17%) the amount of fat in the food chain would be reduced by about 450,000 tonnes, of which 160,000 tonnes would come from livestock (Jones;Undated,p5).

The opportunities to reduce fat vary between animals. With pigs, there has been a tendency over the past 10 years to increase the ratio of lean meat by about 2% per annum - primarily because of changes in consumer taste. Eighty percent of pig carcasses are graded under a Meat and Livestock Commission (MLC) classification scheme and further quality controls operate through the "Charter Quality Scheme" introduced in 1982 (MLC;1986,p1). It is comparatively easy to control the fat content of pigmeat because distribution of fat throughout the carcass makes mechanical separation of the fat a simpler process.

This is not true of cattle and sheep. The reference made by COMA to "carcass grading" applies to the variable premium schemes which operate for cattle and sheep. Under these schemes, grades can be given to animals depending on their fatness and conformation (a guide to the shape and structure of the animal).

The premium paid for the carcass varies according to the grade given. For sheep, there is both an MLC scheme and one used by the EC when carcasses are taken into intervention stores. Each of these schemes, it has been argued, act as: "an incentive to the production of leaner lambs"

(MLC;1986,p4). The MLC scheme only covers 16% of the national flock, but the figures below may give some indication of the spread of the grades.

Table 7.2.   % of Carcasses per MLC Grading-Sheep.

Grade 1	2%	Grade 2	22%
Grade 3l	52%	Grade 3h	18%
Grade 4	5%	Grade 5	1%

Source:MLC;1986,p4.

As you might expect, most animals are bunched in the middle of the scale, primarily in grades 2, 3L and 3H. The Minister of Agriculture:

> ....concluded that it would be appropriate to adjust the certification standards applying under the respective variable premium schemes so as to exclude from eligibility the fatter animals (ie, in the case of cattle those falling into fat class 5; and those covered by the fatter end of the MLC's fat class 4 in the case of sheep (MAFF;1985,p3).

By adjusting the prices that can be obtained in each category, it is possible to use price incentives to encourage farmers to produce animals which fall into lower fat categories. Not all farmers will be affected because many cattle are sold at auction where price "differentiation may not be so apparent" (MLC;1986,p3).

As the system stood before the adjustments were made very few animals fall into the categories that were abolished, perhaps 3% (Personal Correspondence (K);1987). Of course, those that did contributed disproportionately to the amount fat in the food chain. Even so, these carcasses have not necessarily been removed from the food chain altogether - the farmers simply got a lower price for them. The MLC were prepared to sanction the abolition of Grade 4 in sheep fatness but MAFF decided that only the high category of this grade should be removed (Personal Correspondence (K);1986). It seems likely that MAFF was acting on behalf of the NFU when it rejected the MLC proposal, because it would be farmers who had the most to lose from larger penalties in a greater number of grades. As they stand, these changes will still treble the number of carcasses rejected for a premium.

Without wishing to be overly critical, there are still obstacles to the proper implementation of this policy. It is still possible for lean carcasses to be rejected for premium payments because they do not comply with the correct standards of conformation. Jones has argued:

> ...the current system of subsidy payments encourages
> farmers to produce fatter animals and it is time there
> was a re-appraisal of the usefulness of "conformation"
> as an indicator of the value of a carcase
> (Jones;1986,p14).

In short, lean animals may still be rejected for a premium payment because their "conformation" is wrong.

In the case of lambs (or, in Eurospeak, "sheepmeat"), the differences in the premium prices paid in the various grades are not large enough to act as an incentive to farmers to avoid carcasses falling into the highest fat category.

The EEC system of carcass grading, which operates when the carcasses are taken into intervention stores, does encourage the production of leaner carcasses. However, there have been criticisms of the scheme from the meat industry itself because it is the leaner meat which is most likely to be taken into intervention stores, leaving fatter animals on the market (Personal Correspondence (K);1987).

These problems are augmented when you look at farmer's attitudes to politically-led change. Farmers argue they will produce whatever the consumer wants as long as they are given the incentive to do so:

> ...we farmers are businessmen,....with major capital
> assets from which we need to make a profit. That
> means we must react to the needs of our markets...we
> feel even the consumer influence at one step removed
> (French;1986,p24-25).

Their argument is that unless there is a market available, they have no incentive to reduce their fat production simply because governments or health professionals say they should. In the past farmers have been very resistant to change particularly if change has been politically motivated. Minor, incremental adjustments are far more acceptable to producers and manufacturers than are major, overnight changes because they are reversible. Farmers want to avoid a situation in which further changes in consumer preferences (faddism) mean they have mistakenly made changes in breeding, feeding and slaughtering just because the government said it was good for consumers. The financial incentive to farmers may be less useful than expected if it is not supplemented with clear and irreversible attempts to maintain consumer preferences along health lines. This would give farmers the confidence to change. Once again, the need for a policy on dietary change to be "consistent" is self-evident.

The policy problems of adjusting the carcass grading system share much in common with those of food labelling and health education. In each case, the government has retained the same policy makers, the same procedures and the same principles as before and adjusted the COMA recommendations to them. It is, therefore, a very clear example of incremental policy making which has gone as far as it is going to go. In a letter to a consumer group dated 1986 the Minister of Agriculture stated that his Ministry had done all it intended to do on the COMA report (Personal Correspondence (L);1987).

The Common Agricultural Policy (CAP) It is probably best to begin with the official analysis of the role that the CAP plays with regard to diet and health:

> The Government believes that production should be geared to demand as expressed in the market place. In general the commodity regimes of the CAP do not discourage individuals from implementing the COMA dietary recommendations if they wish to do so (MAFF;1985,p4).

This is the official position on the CAP's contribution to COMA's dietary recommendations and it is, of course, consistent with the belief that dietary change should be consumer led.

Approximately 95% of EEC produce is covered by a CAP regime, and the dairy sector has received a disproportionate amount of support (CECG;1984,p7). In 1983, one third of the total CAP budget was spent in this sector, despite a 20% surplus of production over requirements (CECG;1984,p19). Milk production has been subject to support prices which have encouraged production even when demand has been falling. Hence, there are butter mountains and large quantities of liquid milk turned into skimmed milk powder. Dairy products are, perhaps, the most obvious example of how the CAP does not work in the interests of public health. Consider the following:

153

At present, the EC raises the prices of all milk products, and then chooses to subsidize for human consumption the product with the highest fat content (butter), while the skimmed milk products go mainly to the animal population (CECG;1985,p3-4).

To reduce the over-capacity, quotas were set on milk production in 1984 and a penalty was incurred by producers who exceeded their quota (Personal Correspondence (G);1986). Subsequently, quotas appear to have affected smaller dairy farmers very badly and only larger farms have managed to cope with the system.

Whether a restriction of supply discourages healthy eating habits is difficult to establish conclusively. Higher prices discourage consumption of high fat products and so, as far as COMA is concerned, the policy is consistent. However, health is not the primary objective of the policy and the benefits are, at best, coincidental.

There are many other examples where this coincidence, between the goals of dietary change and the CAP, does not exist. Butter is an obvious example. Over 1,000,000 tonnes of butter is held in intervention stores most of which goes to Eastern Europe, but other methods are also used to dispose of it. In the winter of 1986-7, food parcels containing butter were distributed by the EEC through voluntary agencies - a move which was condemned at the time as being contrary to dietary guidelines (Scott;1987,p2). There have also been butter and cheese subsidies available to hospitals and charities, and food manufacturers have been encouraged to use butter instead of other fats - consequently, it has found its way into cakes, confectionary, biscuits and ice cream when it might not otherwise have done so (CECG;1985,p3).

If some policies rest upon an uncomfortable "coincidence", other motives are even more difficult to discern. For example, in 1986 the EC banned farmers from artificially implanting hormones into cattle, a decision which was taken against scientific advice (Gowes and Dawney;1986). While, on the face of it, this appears to be a victory for a consumer lobby opposed to artificial implantation, the decision also benefits the Commission. There is little point in increasing the rate of growth in cattle when the EEC already has too much beef. In short, it is not always clear why EC decisions were made, nor is it possible to know whether the basis of those decisions were compatible with the dietary changes advocated by health professionals.

Meat receives only 12.7% of CAP spending and only beef and veal have intervention and support prices. These tend to keep prices down which is fortuitous because production has been increasing by about 0.5 - 1.0% per annum over the past decade, while consumption has been falling (CECG;1984,p16 and 14). Food manufacturers have to contend with restrictions on meat imports and community preference, which protects EEC producers. Consequently, cheaper imported meat which is suitable for meat products has to be forsaken and this, in turn, raises the price of the manufacturers products. Again, in health terms this may be no bad thing, but the question of how reliable such a policy is still remains. The liberalisation of world trade could stand such a policy on its head. Poultry is another example which, even though it does not generally receive support prices, is still affected by the CAP. The high price of animal feed, and tariffs on cheaper imports mean an increase in costs to poultry farmers at a time when poultry is seen as an alternative to red meat. In this case, the CAP certainly is a disincentive to dietary change if one believes that the price of a good affects the level of its consumption.

One final example will do to illustrate the complexities of the CAP and its relationship to health goals. In 1987, the EC proposed a tax on oils and fats which, it said, was needed to pay for the oilseeds regime. Because Spain and Portugal had oilseed industries and both were about to join the Community, the costs of the regime were likely to rise considerably. In all likelihood this was not the true motive. The tax would raise the price of butter substitutes (eg. margarine), increase butter sales and hence reduce surpluses. Such interference in the market was not appreciated by the food industry (see: FDF;1987, SCOPA;1987, and BCCCA;1987). The Margarine and Shortening Manufacturers Association argued, quite rightly, that the tax would: "...seriously undermine Government dietary policies" (MSMA;1987,p2). Although the British government did oppose the tax, its opposition was based on the market effects of the policy, not its health consequences (Financial Times;1987).

It is not simply that the CAP has not been used to pursue health goals, but the idea itself seems alien to the Foodstuffs division in Brussels:

> It is difficult to see how direct incentives could be given to farmers to respond to dietary goals, but many recent decisions on agricultural policy have been made to adjust supply to demand in a surplus situation.

155

It was further argued that:

> ...by far the most important influence [on the disposal
> of surplus stock] is that of consumer choice (Gray;
> 1986,p14).

Once again, we return to the "consumer-led change" thesis and the preservation, in principle at least, of a competitive market. The insistence on consumer-led change rests very uncomfortably with the operation of the CAP which, to all intents and purposes, does affect consumer choice. The argument that incentives cannot be given to farmers seems odd when farmers are manipulated by the CAP all of the time. What is most "difficult" is to see why there can be incentives for one reason, and not for another. Whether one believes that the CAP should be used to pursue dietary change is a vexed question which rests with our opinions on whether demand should be manipulated for health reasons rather than, as happens at the moment, for supply reasons. A less vexed question is whether the CAP does, or might, act as a disincentive to dietary change, and here the answer is pretty clear. If the British government believes that the CAP does not act as disincentive then this would, of course, explain why it is difficult to find examples of it trying to change the policy in line with the COMA recommendations. The problem appears to be that in this case the British government is wrong.

The position of the European Commission on the COMA report was given in reply to a question from a British MEP, which asked for COMA to be considered on policies concerning oils and fats and some dairy products:

> It is the Commission's opinion that one should view
> some of the recommendations of this report....., with
> some degree of caution. The conclusions drawn by
> many medical experts on this subject, have an inherent
> weakness since often these studies have not been based
> on a sufficiently large test group (CECG;1985,p8).

We are now back to the problem of proof we looked at in Chapter Three. The Commission has roughly the same opinion of the scientific evidence that the British government had in the 1970's. Even if it accepted the COMA report as scientifically valid, this would not mean that the Commission would also accept that the CAP was detrimental to dietary change - indeed, it does not accept this at all.

The British position on the CAP has been far more strongly influenced by the size of the British budget contribution, the cost of the CAP in general and the responsiveness of the various regimes to market forces, than it has to health considerations because it, mistakenly, believes that the CAP presents no obstacles to dietary change.   The evidence suggests that disincentives do exist; that incentives are largely coincidental and vulnerable to change and that the EC shares the consumer-led thesis with the British government. As I said earlier, the point is not necessarily that the CAP should discriminate in favour of dietary change, but rather that it should not discriminate against it.

Critique, Discussion and Conclusion

The response of the British government to the COMA recommendations is consistent with its historical position on other preventive issues. There are two central features to this approach: (1) dietary change should be consumer-led, and (2) the government is responsible for the information which will allow consumers to make informed choices. We saw in the last chapter that this type of approach does have its problems, and most of these are evident here. We also saw that the constraints under which preventive health operates come primarily from protecting the freedom of the individual to choose lifestyles in addition to the economic or commercial consequences of, for example, large scale shifts in consumption patterns. Again, these features have been replicated in the response of the government to the COMA report.

There appear to be good grounds for believing that the policies which emanated from the COMA report are not working as intended. The Royal Society of Medicine (1989) noted that while the incidence of CHD was falling in Britain, the consumption of saturated fat was not. Even in the groups which are most at risk (middle aged men) there has been little change, and the dietary trends in children and young people are not encouraging. The reduction in CHD is the result of changes in exercise and smoking habits, not saturated fat intake:

> Both National Food Survey data and supply side data
> show that this [total energy eaten as fat]
> has.....remained unchanged over the past 10 years at
> about 42%......The COMA report recommended that

fat intake should be around 35% of total energy: Britain is clearly not reaching this target (Rayner;1989,p45).

> The scale of the problem may have been under-estimated at the time the COMA panel reported: The [COMA] Report specified that everybody in Britain should now have the facility for identifying whether they are eating more than 35% fat. But as we discovered over the next year or two, three quarters of the total population of all ages had an intake in excess of 35%...Implementing that upper limit would have induced the most dramatic change in fat intake in this country (James, *in*, Royal Society;1989,p4-5).

Without being unduly pessimistic, this suggests that one of the major risk factors in CHD has remained largely unchanged despite the policies outlined in this chapter. James indicates that the numbers of people who need to modify their diets are greater than first thought, which in turn means that the policies have more work to do.

Of course, this does not mean that the rate of CHD is not falling, but it does mean that the policy to reduce CHD through dietary change is failing. Such a failure is significant not only for the rates of CHD, but also for the prospects for dietary change in general.

If we look at the four elements of a strategy to prevent CHD which were outlined in Chapter Three, this failure becomes understandable, if not inevitable.

A Preventive Strategy While prevention had received much attention in the 1970's, and continues to do so in the 1980's (DHSS;1987, Committee of Public Accounts;1986), CHD has historically been seen as treatable, rather than preventable. The initial professional and political response was technological and the costs to the NHS have been extremely high. The National Audit Office (NAO) noted that the hospital sector absorbs half the cost of treating CHD (£250m) and that the number of by-pass operations quadrupled between 1977 and 1986 (NAO;1989,p22). In comparison to the funds available to prevent the disease, there is an obvious imbalance. No NHS funds have been ear-marked for preventing CHD, all work has to be accommodated within existing budgets. The Look After Your Heart Programme is the only example of special fund being made available besides that which has gone into research. It still seems that the urgency generated by the need for treatment colours perceptions of the most "worthwhile" strategy to combat the disease.

A National Policy Some aspects of the government's response to COMA are national (the food labelling for example), and others are not - counselling those at risk. The National Audit Office (NAO) drew attention to the local variations in approach within the United Kingdom. For example, the DoH does not have comprehensive statistics on the incidence of heart disease:

> the [health] departments do not routinely collect
> comprehensive data on the nature, extent and morbidity
> from the disease...[the sources that are used]...fall short
> of providing a comprehensive picture of the morbidity
> of heart disease, which makes it difficult to assess either
> changes in incidence rates or the effectiveness of control
> measures (NAO;1989,p12).

The National Forum report also said that the absence of quantified targets makes measuring the success (or failure) of the policy very difficult. Similarly, there is very little inter-departmental coordination at the national level:

> Despite repeated calls, there is still no cabinet level
> committee to look at coronary heart disease prevention
> in contrast to the situation for AIDS, drugs and alcohol
> misuse (National Forum;1988,p111).

The comparison with the AIDS and Heroin campaigns is interesting because in these cases the programmes took on the aura of both health education and moral crusade which may account for their prominence. The absence of a cabinet committee on preventing CHD also reflects the historical tendency for the food and health policy areas to be seen as separate entities, discretely pursuing their own policy ends.

If the rationale for a National Strategy is to plan and coordinate resources, or simply to be consistent across the country, then incomplete information and the absence of the machinery to coordinate must be seen as failings of the policy. It is difficult to see how such as strategy could work if disaggregated data is not available and agencies are working independently of each other.

....and Local Level Initiatives Effective local and community action is central to all preventive strategies, whether aimed at CHD or not. The evidence suggests that the ability of health authorities to fulfil the recommendations of COMA are constrained in two ways:

> The DHSS has not made special financial resources available to the District and Regional health Authorities for coronary heart disease prevention, (National Forum; 1988,p106).
>
> ...national strategies have not, thus far, included departmental guidance for health authorities in developing specific programmes aimed at coronary heart disease prevention (NAO;1989,p2).

The DHSS had asked health authorities for information on their initiatives, but this did not provide it with "..sufficient information to enable them to assess the extent of initiatives being undertaken and their integration with Look After Your Heart (NAO;1989,p 16)." The NAO's primary criticism was that at the local level the existence of health promotion in general was sporadic and:

> Generally, the NAO found little evidence of monitoring of the effectiveness of health promotion activities to determine whether there was an awareness and avoidance of coronary heart disease risk factors by the local populations (NAO;1989,p15).

Monitoring and evaluation are often the first aspects of the policy process to go when money is tight (Hogwood and Gunn;1984). Again, this does not mean local initiatives do not exist, but it does mean that they are sporadic and may not occur in the areas of greatest need. Without local policies, the other policies from the COMA report are undermined. In short, local policies to prevent CHD may rely upon the solvency of the health authority, the needs of the population, the ability of the HEA to persuade the authority (or other local agencies/groups) to take on CHD prevention. The process appears to be extremely arbitrary. Local authorities have developed their own food policies and many health authorities have developed similar policies but again, this has been done despite central government rather than because of it. Indeed, one local authority had to abandon plans for a local

160

food policy because it was rate-capped.

The National Policy should be Consistent Much of this, and the previous section, has implicitly dealt with the internal contradictions and inconsistencies of the policies of the past five years. The financial constraints on health and education authorities, the lack of central coordination, the absence of central guidelines to health authorities, the workings of the CAP and the like. There are many other things that could be mentioned which would confirm these contradictions and inconsistencies. The Royal Society of Medicine report highlights the ambiguity of the government's position on the COMA report:

> **Anne Dillon** said that Civil Servants had been anxious to point out that the COMA Report overall had been accepted by the government. But that did not mean that it accepted each of its recommendations, which had potentially massive long-term effects across the whole range of Government (Dillon, in, Royal Society;1989,p19).

This, of course, makes evaluating the consistency of the policies very difficult. Which of the COMA recommendations have the government accepted? The "massive long-term effects" are, presumably, those on industry and we have seen in this chapter and others that this has qualified much of what MAFF and the DoH have done. Assuming that a concern for the economic consequences of policy is legitimate, we are drawn back to the idea consumer-led change, in which consumer sovereignty in the market place, rather than the state, determines the food on sale. But, here too, the approach is not coi...stent. The bottom line of the "lifestyle approach" to preventive medicine has always been that the state provides information upon which individuals make their own choices. Yet, we saw with the food labelling regulations, the NACNE report, the JACNE leaflet and the report on the diets of school children that the information to assist informed dietary change has not been forthcoming. A vicious circle is created in which changes will occur in some areas (ie. the development and consumption of "health" products), but will not occur in other, more mainstream products. In turn, this will not provide the incentive for manufacturers to change their mainstream products, and hence consumer-led change may become an anomaly. As the National Forum report argued, it is the mainstream products which are the most important, and yet, the most unlikely to change:

> To deal with nutritionally-based health problems we
> need to improve the mainstream products which people
> eat most of the time. With the exception of the
> reduction of salt in bread and soups, this has not
> generally been the industries' approach (National
> Forum;1988,p72).

A lifestyle approach, which relies upon consumers leading dietary change, should not be taken to mean there is no role for the state. Even if such an approach could work, it implies that state agencies have much to do in informing the public of the choices that are available to them. Lower socio-economic groups are particularly vulnerable in this respect and yet the only concession to socio-economic variables is the "Look After Your Heart" programme which targets those groups.

Again, it is difficult to escape the conclusion that there is a high degree of inconsistency in the response to the COMA recommendations. If an effective anti-coronary strategy should provide the opportunity for consumers to change their diets and, wherever possible, remove obstacles to their doing so, then it must be argued that so far the policy has been ineffective. It must also be said that it is at odds with the historically accepted role of the state in providing information and education to consumers.

A Population and an At Risk Approach The strategies adopted to encourage dietary change and reduce CHD have had a "population" and an "at risk" component. Each however, has been severely qualified by their effects on pre-existing policies or other political priorities. This is most noticable with food labelling and other policies coming from MAFF. Here all the historical, ideological and institutional blocks to dietary change which were anticipated in Chapter Five have materialised. The population element of the policy on CHD are , therefore, so qualified as to be of little utility in promoting dietary change. Given the role of preventive medicine in the past, perhaps a vigorous "at risk" approach would be more likely given the state's pre-disposition toward protecting the vulnerable. Here again, however, even the strategy which might be thought the most manageable has had its limitations. Health promotion struggles under the conflicting policy goals of comprehensive monitoring on the one hand and resource constraints on the other. Autonomous local inititiatives tussle with nationally prescribed funding arrangements for local authorities and health authorities. Despite the fact that Britain has the institutional arrangements to provide an effective "at risk" strategy it has neither the resources or the ideological commitment from the centre to make it work. The fact that two strategies are available does not mean that either will work without central support. It is clear that both COMA and the government knew each approach was necessary yet neither has been fully implemented as COMA suggested or as any policy might be expected to be implemented.

*   *   *   *   *

It is, perhaps, too easy to criticise governments. They all have to make decisions which are unpopular and have never yet devised a perfect policy on anything. What makes the politics of dietary change interesting is the discrepancy between the stated intentions of governments and their actions. Should this be put down to ineptitude, design, necessity or a combination of the three? Or, perhaps, it has nothing to do with governments at all?

One of the striking aspects of the debate over dietary change has been the degree to which elite professionals have been politically active, for example, in establishing the Coronary Prevention Group and the National Forum for Coronary Heart Disease Prevention. Their ability to place the issue on the political agenda is not in question - what is questionable is their ability to continue to influence policy implementation and outcomes once they have forced action from the government. This is all the more evident in the case of the ordinary professionals, whose power is all the more concentrated within the NHS.

With the possible exception of smoking, which was the subject of a BMA campaign in 1984, the promotion of health issues has not been a feature of professional organisations. The 1976 report by the Royal College of Physicians and the British Cardiac Society was an important document in medical terms yet, once the report was published, there was no follow-up by those responsible for it. They perceived their role as simply disseminating information to their readers, not encouraging the practical changes advocated. It was the failure of elite professionals to take this lead which prompted others to set up the Coronary Prevention Group as a campaigning organisation. Similarly, the 1986 BMA report called upon the government to change some of its agricultural policies. Again however, once the report had been published, a conscious decision was taken not to pursue the subject any further (Personal Correspondence (N);1988).

Given that it is elite professionals who are primarily responsible for

163

articulating the views of the profession as a whole (either as experts or representatives), the absence of such articulation important:

> **Anne Dillon** said that...One of the main problems with medical attitudes was that there was a lack of strong leadership and insufficiently firm statements from those people qualified to make them.
> ...those who wished to bring about change had shown a remarkable naivety about the way that change was instituted. It was not enough for the British Cardiac Society and the Royal College of Physicians to produce reports. Unless there was a constituency to promote such information, nothing would happen (Dillon, *in*, Royal Society;1989,p17-18).

Thus, while there has been a broad agreement among elite professionals concerning diet and CHD, professionals operating within the NHS have not been targeted by the elite. More importantly, however, the professional politicisation of the policy area has come primarily from concerned individuals, rather than from established organisations. Clearly this is a much weaker political position for those who are advocating changes in diets and may well account for why many general practitioners do not take the medical evidence as seriously as might be expected.

So, professionals have not adopted a politically effective strategy. Nevertheless, this cannot be the whole story, because the COMA panel were *invited* to make recommendations to government which were subsequently only partially implemented. So, we have to look elsewhere to understand the discrepancy between stated intention and action.

A large part of the explanation lies in the historical characteristics of the food and health policy area. Even if the DoH had been firmly committed to a vigorous anti-coronary policy, many of the recommendations of the COMA panel were aimed at MAFF. Historically MAFF has enjoyed almost total autonomy and control over policy making, but this control has been based upon certain assumptions about the role of the state in the food supply and the legitimacy of commercial interests - it has seldom intervened on the demand side of food, except in times of food scarcity. The recommendations of COMA have disturbed these assumptions which appear to rest upon the twin principles of (1) retaining the competitiveness of food manufacturing and (2) the sovereignty of the consumer - principles it shares with the DoH. Hence, when MAFF came to devise a food labelling system it was not only health considerations which were its guiding principle, but the effects that the labels would have on the competitiveness of industry. The recommendations of COMA were very difficult to accommodate in the cultural context within which MAFF makes its decisions. This has been compounded by the fact that consumer and professional representation within MAFF has never been strong. Thus, the opportunities for interests other than those associated with food and farming to challenge the existing orthodoxy within MAFF is minimal. For MAFF, then, the responses do not bear the hallmarks of ineptitude because they are predictable. Rather, the actions of MAFF are a combination of those things which have to be done, and those ways of doing things which are preferred.

The DoH has also had constraints under which it had to work. The strength of the curative ideology has played some part in the differentials between curative and preventive expenditure and can also account, in part at least, for professional organisations focussing their attention on the NHS rather than on the environment which creates ill-health. Equally, however, there is far less political mileage in having an effective preventive strategy than in performing by-pass operations.

It, too, has had to contend with the possible economic consequences of its actions, by qualifying the advice it has given to consumers. The dietary change debate is pushing for a more active role from the DoH, while the DoH is struggling with its traditional, hands off, role toward the population. Preventive medicine has historically been aimed primarily at the vulnerable and there has been a discernible reluctance on the part of the DoH to change this, despite the obvious need to do so.

In addition there are the more idiosyncratic features of the governments of the 1980's which have had an ideological distaste for extending the role of the state or spending more money than they deemed absolutely necessary. Again, the tendency is not to favour an "ineptitude" explanation. It is difficult to escape the conclusion that the apparent degree of ineptitude, as noted by the National Audit Office and the National Forum Report, has to be deliberate. Technically, a strategy which neither specifies an overall objective or a means to achieving change is in serious danger of not qualifying as a policy at all (Hogwood and Gunn; 1984, Ham and Hill;1984). While there are identifiable strategies (means) their effectiveness has been qualified by ideological and commercial factors.

In short, it is not difficult to see why the COMA report was accepted - the political costs of not doing so would have been great. On this rests much of the explanation for the apparent ineffectiveness of the responses to the COMA report, because the job still remains of implementing the recommendations that were accepted. Here is the real test of quite how serious a government is prepared to be about dietary change.

8 Theoretical Explanations

For most of this study, the theoretical tools and the empirical evidence have been kept separate. I have tried to provide an empirical account of the politics of dietary change, but this can do little more than explain in the particular. Yet the concepts of networks and communities, structure and agency should apply to all policy making and so offer the opportunity to generate new hypothesese about the way we are governed, and what we can expect from our polity.

This chapter, then, applies the concepts which were first mentioned in Chapter Two, to what is known about the politics of dietary change. It is particularly concerned to look at how networks and communities work, because it has seemed that they perform what can best be described as a control and defence function for public policy - they are not simply there for the convenience of policy makers. But networks need to be married to something else, something which can accommodate agency and the peculiarities of structures, and this is also an important task of this chapter. Finally, I want to look at the structural role of capital and to see how the interpretation used here, differs from that found in the pluralist literature.

Policy Communities, Networks and Explanations

In Chapter Two I argued that the political relationships in MAFF and the DOH could be characterised as communities and networks. The first job of this chapter is to establish whether policy communities and networks actually provide a good description of these relationships.

Since the Second World War there have been persistent political relationships within MAFF. MAFF's relationship with the farmers is the easiest of all to characterise because of this continuity. During and after the war, agricultural policies were formulated almost exclusively between MAFF and the NFU and this relationship has persisted even through the trauma of British entry into the EEC. While there is some evidence to suggest that there is now less common ground between MAFF and the NFU than there used to be, it is nevertheless true that this relationship remains strong. According to the criteria laid down in Chapter Two, this is a policy community, and Smith agrees (1988,1989) [1].

It is the agricultural policy community which has been dominant within MAFF during the post-war period and has provided constraints under which other policy areas have operated. But, this is not the only policy community that the NFU belongs to, because at the sub-sectoral level they clearly have an input into decisions on, for example, meat and meat manufacturing.

The case of the food industry presents a more complicated picture, because the industry is extremely diverse. Nevertheless, it appears as though policy communities do exist in key areas. In the dairy sector this revolves around the Joint Committee of the Milk Marketing Board and the Dairy Trade Federation; for meat it includes the Bacon and Meat Manufacturers Association, the Meat and Livestock Commission, the NFU and MAFF. It is these interests, above others, which have the strongest input into policy. Equally, it is possible to identify not only a high level of

---

[1] The membership has been stable through time; there is clearly a field of authority and responsibility (agricultural policy); there is a consensus on policy values which revolve around state support for agriculture and the maximisation of production; relations are asymmetric to the extent that MAFF does have the last word and there has been the exclusion of alternative opinions in decision making, notably those of consumers.

integration (which denotes the existence of policy communities), but other characteristics of these communities as well, for example, shared policy values (promotion and continued competitiveness of the sub-sectors); the exclusion of those who challenge those values (unless on the details rather than the substance, of policy) and, again, a predominant role for MAFF. In these two important sub-sectors, therefore, it is possible to find integrated structures which are central to the decision making in their respective policy areas. This is not to say that they are unresponsive to other values which exist outside of the policy community, but rather, that they interact with these interests largely on their own terms. The changes in the carcass grading system and food labelling were a very good examples of this.

If these sub-sectors are reasonably discrete, there are certain issues which cross sub-sectoral boundaries and touch upon values which are common across policy areas. Food labelling is one such issue, as would be compositional standards for foods. In these cases, it is not sub-sectoral policy communities which are responsible for making decisions, but the network of interests which revolve around this particular issue (an issue network). An issue such as labelling, which affects so much of the food industry, will generate a greater homogeneity of purpose even within such a diverse industry. The network is dominated by producers even though the issue itself has given greater opportunities for alternative values to be heard through consultations with, for example, consumer groups. Despite the fact that issue networks are more open arenas, the food industry still shares certain values with MAFF and still has greater structural resources than its competitors. It is not difficult to see that even with an issue such as food labelling which is more competitive than, say, agricultural policy, some interests are simply better placed than others to influence policy.

It is quite clear that a network did develop around the issue of food labelling, and that it had done so before the COMA report was published. Indeed, MAFF had just completed its work on amending the 1955 Food and Drug Act before it began work on the COMA recommendations.

It seems fair to argue that the pervasive presence of food and farming interests in, or near, MAFF should not be ignored. There are producer networks which services various policy communities, issues networks and sub-sectoral networks in terms of clientele, service provision to its members etc. On some issues there will be conflict between these various sub-sectors and they will withdraw into their own respective networks - this happened with food irradiation when some parts of industry were in favour (particularly those dealing with fresh food) and some were not (for example, those who "froze" food).

Technocrats can be found in three places - within the Scientific division of MAFF, within the Food and Drink Federation or the associations which comprise the FDF, and in the British Nutrition Foundation. They comprise a *technocratic network* which services both MAFF and the food industry more generally. As this network services its parent organisations it reinforces the values of their policy communities and networks by providing scientific legitimacy to their policies. In other words, the technocratic network espouses a consistent world view which argues for a balanced diet and asserts the basic soundness of the food supply. This fits very well with the broader values of competition and innovation that are to found elsewhere in the food industry. Once again, this network should be seen as a network in its own right and as a resource for other policy communities and networks. In Wilks and Wright's terms, it is a policy community itself: a pool of technocrats.

Historically, these networks and communities continue unless the food supply itself is threatened, then, the number of interests which have a meaningful input into policies within MAFF increases. New policy communities are created which are more consumer orientated, and technocratic and scientific networks are elevated in terms of their political input into policy and broadened in terms of the pool of experts from which they are drawn. In short, MAFF has found ways of servicing itself and dealing with its own policy problems by drawing in those interests which have things it wants.

The primary source of professional power is the NHS where their resources are valued and their position dominant - though less so than in the past perhaps. Rhodes' contention that professionals within the NHS can be seen as a professionalised network is reasonable because they have a pervasive presence, fairly uniform interests and a pretty consistent effect throughout the NHS. Policy communities exist within health authorities, and within the DoH itself (for example the Units of Nutrition, Preventive Medicine and Heart Disease). In addition, there are elite networks which may be representational (eg. the BMA) or advisory elites which service the DoH - COMA is one of these. So, we have to distinguish between the professionalised network of the NHS, policy communities within the DoH and the elite networks. Conspicuous by its absence is a network which is firmly rooted in all or part of MAFF.

There is evidence to suggest, however, that technocrats within MAFF have penetrated the decision making structures of the DoH and extended the technocratic element in policy. For example, there were MAFF observers on the NACNE committee, the JACNE committee and the 1984 COMA

170

panel. In each of these cases, the observers did make a contribution to policies.

In purely descriptive terms, there are two discrete policy areas offering various resources to their members but interacting only occasionally. Within these policy boundaries there are more complex patterns of political relationships.

Professionals have not been in a position to alter the scientific basis of food policies because of their structural location and because MAFF has been wedded to the old nutritional orthodoxy. This puts the prime movers of dietary change in no better position (politically) to influence the government than anyone else.

If health professionals are not members of the communities and networks of MAFF that make policy, then their opportunities to influence policy reside in their attempts to influence the political environment within which decisions are made. They are only different to other groups in terms of the resources that they bring with them. Elites and professionals have the capacity to make the state incur political costs by highlighting the inadequacies of public policy and/or its health consequences. All interests in this environment try to accumulate political resources, either by generating new ones (eg. enlarging group membership) or taking resources from opponents (eg. influencing the media presentation of issues). This has been the strategy adopted by individuals and ad hoc groups of professionals and has been particularly noticeable in their creation of the Coronary Prevention Group and their media work.

In the last chapter I argued that even though certain elite professionals have been involved in this process their peak organisations (the BMA and the Royal College of Physicians) have not tended to become involved to the same extent. They have treated the issue as though it were one which *could* be resolved within the NHS, that is, they have published reports for professionals to read as though that, in itself, could resolve the problem of diet and heart disease. The efficacy of professional influence has been reduced as the peak organisations retained the pre-existing policy orientations of the networks they were involved in.

Accumulating political resources allows groups to manipulate, to their advantage, their relationships with decision makers. Of course, anyone can try to do this, not only those who are opposed to present policies. Indeed, Lindblom argued that the resources available to business were partly applied in policy environments, and partly within decision making structures (1977,Chap.14). In turn this means that those who have structural advantages in the first place, will be better placed to retain them.

Having said this, professionals and other groups have managed to politicise the issue of dietary change in the one way which was almost guaranteed to provoke a response from the state, that is, to call into question the state's ability to secure an adequate supply of food.

If this external environment has diverse, competing interests now, what about the "internal environments" which make decisions? Well, we can tell quite a lot about these by looking at the policies themselves.

There are a number of persistent features of MAFF's policies which are central to the paradigm within which policies are made. Certainly since WWII these appear to be (1) state support for agriculture, (2), minimal controls on the products presented for sale (once safety and integrity have been assured), (3) non-interference in the demand side of the market as far as (1) and (2) will allow, and (4) no unnecessary restrictions on the innovative or competitive abilities of suppliers in the market. In times of food scarcity, it is (3) and (4) which appear to change most, either through simple food shortages or through price manipulation. These characteristics of food policy effectively determine the membership of policy communities within MAFF, and also the membership of the networks.

But there is also a scientific paradigm as well which reinforces policy by supplying a rational scientific justification for policies which focuses on individual choice from the foods available. The paradigm is a cognitive one (Laffin;1986). It is made up of both scientific knowledge and a set of values to which members of the community adhere, but should not be confused with "rules of the game" which are simply the terms of engagement. So, values and science, at least on an abstract level, can become indistinguishable. Of course, this applies as much to those who oppose policies, as it does to those who don't.

The paradigm excludes some interests straightaway - others have to abide by the rules of the game, even though they are ideologically opposed to the paradigm. Either way, the entry qualifications are stiff. The Consumers Association, which has members on the Food Advisory Committee, has been criticised for not taking a more active role in "selling" dietary change to MAFF, but believes it would compromise the access to decision making centres they already have (Personal Correspondence (Q); 1986). In other words, access is dependent upon accepting the rules, if not the values, of the networks and communities that exist.

The internal environment of the DoH rest upon other assumptions all of which are consistent with the role that MAFF has in the food supply: (1), preventive medicine relied in large part on individual responsibility; (2), the state can advise on, but not direct, individual lifestyles; (3), the state

172

extends this role only to those who are "vulnerable" physically or financially. There is nothing in these assumptions that suggests there should be any conflict between MAFF and the DoH unless, of course, the DoH extends its preventive role.

The model of policy communities and networks I gave in Chapter Two suggests that when politicisation occurs we would expect networks and policy communities to manipulate the political tension between themselves and their external environments (depoliticise the issue) while retaining the core values upon which present policies were based. The extent to which networks would be able to do this would depend, in large part, upon their degree of integration, that is, how well they controlled the policy area. What we know of the actions of MAFF and the DoH suggest that this characterisation is the correct one. It is clear that; the intention was to reinstate a consensus; that relations were asymmetric because the last word fell to state agents; the issues raised were confined to particular policy areas and not extended beyond the scope of the report even though such an extension was implied by the report itself; and that certain values were effectively excluded from policy. In short, this amounts to damage limitation and self defence.

The political compatibility between the structures I have outlined so far, and the interests they affect rests upon the ability of policy communities or networks to comply with or control their perceived interests and resources. The persistence of particular policies for a long time implies either a broad consensus on policy, or, the manipulation of the relationships by those with the resources to do so.

Policy change, therefore, comes from shifts in resources and changes in perceptions which, in turn, alter the balance of forces within the structure - in our case, MAFF. In other words, once people perceive a problem with the food supply, then things begin to move.

While the food supply was not perceived as causing public health problems, then a broad consensus did exist. The balance resources shifted very gradually through time because of the normal operation of the structures themselves, that is, post-war policies and production techniques. So, the attempts by MAFF and DoH to prevent the publication of the NACNE report, for example is an attempt to prevent the redistribution of resources from central government agencies to interests within the external environment. In Chapter Two I called this ideological exclusion.

This argument appears to assume that there is no coincidence of interests between MAFF, the food industry and consumers, but it would be an over-simplification to say this. Dietary change creates new product opportunities

173

in the form of "healthy" foods, so to this extent there is a coincidence, but large scale dietary change also implies the loss of existing markets. It is this loss which is the main problem for food manufacturers.

So, we end up with a mixture of intended and unintended consequences. Clearly, competition between groups is a deliberate purposive act and strategies to gain or retain political resources fall into the same category. But there is more to it than this. Firstly, we know that "diseases of affluence" are, in part, the unintended consequences of past policies. Secondly, we also know that policies and political relationships (structures) can become "anchored" - I have called these anchors standardised expressions - towards certain policies rather than others. The creation of these anchors is deliberate, but their effects may not be - witness surplus production and the Common Agricultural Policy. Thirdly, there are actions which have unintended, although predictable, outcomes. These apply to the operation of the market and its effects on consumption.

Knowing that power is the product of resources and that it is exercised through structures adds to network theory certain, necessary, explanatory variables. Without this, we can plausibly argue (hypothesise) that networks and communities will behave in certain ways, but to know how they do it, or what prompts them to it requires some account of agency and resource change.

State and Societal Forces

In this section I want to consider some of the broader structural features of the food and health debate and to look at some of the macro-level variables which are important. These will mostly involve the relationship of the state to capital, primarily because the empirical evidence suggests it is significant. It will be a necessarily brief exercise but will, I hope, add another aspect to the overall explanation.

The evidence suggests that MAFF and industry have a very close relationship which rests upon their coincidence of interests. Does this mean that MAFF has lost the ability to act autonomously? Skocpol (1985) has argued that the tendency has been within political science over the past 15 years or so to emphasise the role of the state as a complex political actor which has the capacity and motive for autonomous action:

> ...state autonomy is not a fixed structural feature of any
> governmental system. It can come and go...the very

174

structural potential for autonomous state action changes
over time, as the organisations of coercion and
administration undergo transformations both internally
and in their relations with societal groups and to
representative parts of government (Skocpol;1985,p14).

This fits nicely with the concepts I have used so far. Again, we get the
impression of gradual structural change through time and the interaction
(mutual adjustment) of the state with groups. We should, according to
Skocpol, attribute some autonomy to state actions, that is, we should expect
the state to have interests of its own and be able to pursue them
independently of other interests. Equally, we should expect this autonomy
to vary through time - sometimes the state will be more reliant upon these
interests than others.

The state clearly has extraordinary responsibilities and resources which
differentiate it, at times, from capital interests and which suggest that it
must be granted autonomy within any theoretical framework. While
explanations of state behaviour will not be found without reference to its
relationship with capital, neither will they be found with reference to these
alone. So, I would also argue that the state cannot be considered as just
another group (see Richardson and Jordan;1979), neither, for that matter, is
capital (see Vogel;1987); policy outcomes have been far too consistently in
favour of capital for this to be the case.

Although it would be wrong to see the power of capital interests as
deterministic, it is clear that it does have certain advantages over the other
groups, and over state agencies as well. This study indicates that there are
four sources of such advantage:

1. *An ideological compatibility between the values and goals of the state,
and those of economic (capital) interests; in our case, food manufacturers
and farmers.* There a particular historical reasons why this is true of food,
and it may not be so of other manufacturing sectors.

Historically, state support for agriculture has been based upon political,
strategic and economic imperatives and has led to substantial state
intervention because the state perceives its best interests to be served in that
way. Policies in this area have, therefore, been far more pragmatic than is
the case for the food manufacturing sector which has not needed such
intervention. As Gamble has argued:

So firmly embedded..[has]...liberal political economy
become that it has rarely appeared a crusading doctrine

in England, but generally as an orthodoxy emanating
from the very bowels of the state (Gamble;1986,p129).

This orthodoxy has been evident in, for example, the permeating influence
of "freedom of choice" which I mentioned earlier. Clearly, it is in the
interests of food manufacturers to be as unrestricted as possible, and this is
a view they share with MAFF. An "advantage" accrues to them because
the recommendations of health professionals and consumer groups are
directed toward greater state intervention in the market, particularly on the
demand side. In short, there is no ideological compatibility between these
recommendations and the historical position of MAFF on intervention in
food manufacturing.

2. *The constraints that the existence of a market in food places upon the
policy options available.* This is the same type of constraint that Ingham
recognised when speaking of the structural position of finance capital in the
first Wilson government:

> The City's unregulated global operations and sterling's
> role placed real constraints on the range of domestic
> policy options by means of the ever present threat of the
> collapse of the currency (Ingham;1984,p215).

This is not to say that the City overtly threatened the government with the
collapse of sterling, but rather, that sterling may have collapsed simply
because of the way the currency markets respond to political and economic
indicators.

Similar constraints present themselves to MAFF. The fact that MAFF
relies upon a free market to supply food implies further that the ability of
that market to fulfil this function must be retained. Certain policy options
are, therefore, ruled out because the existence of the market acts as a
constraint.

These are particularly noticeable in the relationship between the food and
health policy areas. Health policy options in the preventive field have been
constrained by the market implications of recommending population-level
dietary changes. While the state has accepted the need to treat the
vulnerable sections of the population as a special case and to give them
advice and help, to do the same for the whole population would mean large-
scale shifts in consumption patterns which would have severe commercial
repercussions. Without a further commitment to price manipulation,

176

changes in agricultural subsidies and strong, effective health education and information, the worry for MAFF was that the market, which is the only means of food supply and distribution, would have been severely disrupted, prices would have risen sharply in the short term and public confidence in the food supply would have sunk. These are almost unthinkable costs to incur voluntarily. Again, this constitutes an advantage for economic interests because it is not a constraint which can be attributed to other interests in this policy area.

3. *The resources available to farmers and food manufacturers which they can use, or threaten to use, in pursuit of their preferred policies*. The basis of Lindblom's argument rested on the idea that it was the structural constraints of the market and the lobbying of business which makes business "uniquely privileged" (1977,p179). It is this feature of business which is usually focussed on by pluralist interpretations of power in general and the power of groups in particular. In our case, then, what are these resources? Certainly industry's ability to draw on technocratic resources is one and applies both in its dealings with MAFF and the work it does in the external environment of the policy area. Similarly, the financial and organisational resources of industry have been used in, for example, its opposition to the proposed oils and fats tax of the EC, and, of course, in various campaigns to retain sales in areas affected by the COMA recommendations. Equally, Cannon (1987) argued that the food and drink industry had many allies in the House of Commons who have been used to keep up the pressure on the government to re-state publicly its policy commitments and to distance itself from suggested, radical, dietary change. In these respects, industry, and indeed, farmers, can be seen as bearing significant resources over and above those enjoyed by opposing groups.

4. *The costs incurred by the state of not deferring to (3), or attempting to alter (2)*. This differs from the other advantages inasmuch as the state may *want* to do something but cannot afford to do it even though the action itself is possible. One would expect that these types of costs would occur primarily when the state relied upon economic interests to implement certain aspects of policy, or when financial or political costs to the state would be incurred if a certain course of action were taken. In other words, one would expect all structural changes to involve some shift in resources, but under these particular circumstances, the shift away from the state, or toward other interests is seen by the state to be too great.

This type of cost (or resource shift) can take a number of forms, some more tangible than others. For example, the Food and Drink Federation (FDF) has recently established a food intolerance data-bank which gives details of the foods which may cause allergic reactions in consumers (Feedback;1987,p1). Arguably, the cost of such a venture, or one which was similar, would have fallen to MAFF had the FDF not taken the initiative on its own behalf. Similarly, a great deal of the regulation surrounding food, particularly on compositional standards, is voluntary and relies upon the good will of industry. Again, in the absence of this good will, MAFF would incur the cost of having to legislate. The Chief Medical Officer of the DoH (Acheson) gave another example quoted earlier. He said that the government was in a difficult position when promoting dietary changes because such a policy could also promote unemployment in certain industries. Again, under some political circumstances this could be perceived as an unacceptable political cost. This is not to say that the state, or parts of it, cannot be perceived as acting against economic interests, only that to do so may be costly.

This account of the power and advantages of economic interests does differ from those to be found elsewhere, particularly amongst pluralist and neo-pluralist views on capital/state relations. Certainly, orthodox pluralist conceptions of the state (in which I exclude Lindblom) suffer now from problems which have been highlighted by this case study. The first is that there is too little consideration of the difference in power resources available to groups which may skew political outcomes consistently in favour of some groups rather than others. Secondly, they assume that the state has few interests of its own; this is obviously inaccurate given the material I have presented here. And thirdly, pluralist's characterisations of the state assume a clear separation of the state and civil society; without this, the state cannot be seen as independent of the interests of groups, nor can it retain the impartiality necessary for a pluralist polity. As Held points out (Held;1989,p283), without this separation it is difficult, if not impossible, for there to be democratic government in any meaningful sense of the word. Although Smith (1990) has rightly pointed out that pluralists have been unfairly criticised in the past, it is still the case that the framework does not fit the evidence of this study.

Neo-pluralists have not fared a great deal better. Lindblom concedes that "business" is privileged (as Dahl eventually did, Held;1989,p202) but his analysis of the relationship between the state and business is itself flawed both methodologically and theoretically. As Stones observes (1988), there is little mileage in simply finding, as Lindblom does, examples which suggest that the state works in the interests of capital, because there will always be counter-examples which can be forwarded by others to contest arguments presented in this way.

Theoretically, Lindblom goes some way to ameliorating this by making the distinction between "grand" and "secondary" issues, that is, those issues over which business is "uniquely privileged" (grand) and those which are contestable (secondary). While Vogel, in his critique of Lindblom, is unfair in his cursory dismissal of the grand issues Lindblom forwards it is nevertheless true that this sort of approach is very problematic. From the arguments given above, it is clear that ideological commitments are an important explanatory variable, and yet, there is little consideration of this in Lindblom's analysis. Thus, while the pluralist literature can give an account of the overt application of political resources, and neo-pluralists positions recognise some of the constraints and costs that are attributable to economic interests, there is, nevertheless, some explanatory distance between their account of power and advantages, and my own.

On this basis I would argue that the position I have taken is a reasonable one. It does not rely upon the fact that the state has no other interests besides retaining a competitive market. It is perfectly possible, on my analysis, for the state not to act in the interests of capital if it has other interests which conflict with those of capital and which can force it to incur unacceptable costs; indeed, this is a primary source of power for health professionals. Similarly, it does not rely on the state having few interests of its own, independent of capital, for it is clear that the responsibility of maintaining the supply of food lies with the state in the final analysis. Equally, it can account for the obvious ideological compatibility between the state and business, and the constraints which the market places upon the actions of the state, without having to argue that the state is always constrained to act in the interests of capital. In short, to characterise the relationship between the state and capital it is necessary to account for both the consistencies through time (a point which is largely ignored by Vogel) and the inconsistencies (a point which is difficult to explain solely at the empirical level). There is no reason to suppose that the same rules and ideological orientation apply throughout the many decision making centres of the state. We might expect change to be occurring within structures constantly, given that mutual adjustment is happening all the time, but we would not expect the changes to be the same in every structure, as we would not expect all structures to be identical, or even similar.

Most of the sectors of the state, most of the time, are discrete and autonomous to some extent in their everyday operation; besides the competition for resources, there is little overlap between education and defence, for example. It is only when one sector impinges on another - when there is a conflict of interests between sectors - that it is possible to see what the "bottom line" might be for the state more generally.

Conclusion

The key feature of this case study has been the change in the scientific orthodoxy surrounding diet and health. Since WWII many policies and political relationships had been built upon the assumption that if the state had a role to play in the nutritional well-being of the population, it rested upon preventing food scarcity.

Consequently, there developed separate political structures to deal with separate political problems. Within MAFF, policies relating to food and agriculture came to be made in dominant and sub-ordinant policy communities, and networks developed which were primarily the preserve of farmers and food manufacturers. The value bases of these communities and networks revolved around state support for agriculture and non-intervention in the market place, particularly on the demand side.

Health care developed within a discrete system, as might be expected of a predominantly curative system. Hence, problems of health, and the broader social problems attached to vulnerability could be dealt with by the professionalised network which extended to small policy communities in the DoH and to elite representational and advisory networks.

Structural processes (mutual adjustment, the creation of standardised expressions, uneven distribution of resources) kept these structures anchored within their respective policy orientations despite the fact that the scientific basis for food policies and the role implied for nutrition in preventive medicine had changed dramatically.

It has been the ability of MAFF to control policies on food and health and to retain the previous paradigm that has prevented change, and this has been possible because of its command, not only of its own decision making processes, but also of the DoH's as well. Explanations, therefore, come from an account of the resources available and the perceived interests of those within affected structures. If perceptions change as a result of the inherent movements in structures then we can assess both the basis' for policies themselves and the political relationships and values which may wish to protect the policies. So, when we plot changes in policies or describe rules of game and paradigms or argue that food manufacturers are influential we need to establish precisely what it is that is providing the rules, ideology or paradigm. The role of capital (at a macro-level) has to be incorporated because it is a genuine source of many of these variables and we cannot understand the problems of dietary change without reference to them.

9 Conclusion

Politically, the status of food is ambiguous. On the one hand, food has always been a marketed commodity and, as such, it has had both a commercial and a nutritional value. Historically, this has been a crucial aspect of nutrition policy, because of the state's reluctance to interfere in the workings of the market place. This was vividly displayed for the first two years of WWI, when it was believed that, even during war, the market should be allowed to operate freely wherever possible. Once intervention was inevitable extraordinary lengths were gone to in order to protect trading secrecy and fair competition. This same philosophy underpins the state's position on diet and health in the 1980's. Successive governments have argued that changes in consumption have to be consumer led and that the state cannot, or will not, interfere in the workings of the market and direct consumption or supply on health grounds.

On the other hand, food is essential to life and its provision is required regardless of the commercial competence of the consumer. Clearly, there have been times when this dual status has presented conflicts - when the market has been unable to provide for the nutritional needs of the population. I have given the examples of the two world wars and the depression of the 1930's to illustrate this point. At these times the state has directed consumption and become more prominent in the market through price incentives, subsidies, price guarantees etc. Having said this, these were times when there was a threat to food supply for the whole population or large parts of it, and as such are atypical. Before WWII, the state, particularly the Ministry of Health, was reluctant to admit that the market was far less competent in supplying food than it might be. As Boyd-Orr demonstrated, malnutrition was endemic, rather than extraordinary.

After WWII this situation was formally recognised, and the distinction between those who were "vulnerable", in nutritional terms, and those who were not, became the gauge of whether the state supported them either financially or nutritionally. In comparison to pre-WWII Britain this was clearly a major step forward because it not only recognised that the vulnerable were a permanent fixture of British society, but it further committed the British state to an important, though limited, role in supporting them.

Having said this, there are two points which must qualify how far the changes that occurred after WWII represent a step toward the type of policies that health professionals have argued for with diet and heart disease. The first is that there remained a clear distinction between the workings of the system of food supply (ie. the market) and the nutritional intervention of the state. Although the state encouraged food production, this was never done because it would improve the health of the population. Similarly, food manufacture was not directed or encouraged to provide particular foods, only to standardise products. Secondly, and as a corollary to this, health professionals have never had a great deal of influence over food supply beyond establishing what is immediately dangerous to health and what is not. Even then, expert input into policies has been extremely technocratic in nature. The compatibility between the nature of the food supply and the nutritional orthodoxy of the post-WWII period meant that this situation was acceptable politically both to professionals or the state, because such nutritional problems as did exist were confined, once again, to the vulnerable sections of the population.

This would have mattered less if the structure and organisation of the preventive medical services were orientated toward the whole population. Again, however, these services are primarily directed toward the vulnerable, and very little of their work is directed toward educating and informing everyone.

It is not difficult to see, therefore, that when diet and CHD became a political issue in the 1980's there were a great many structural and ideological constraints on, what might be deemed by the state, as acceptable policy initiatives. Food production and supply had seldom had a health component, state interference in the market had little historical precedent, professionals were not well placed politically to influence the formulation and implementation of policy and the preventive services were primarily orientated toward the vulnerable.

When the issue did reach the political agenda, three other factors compounded these structural and ideological problems. The first relates back to the assertion that dietary changes should be consumer led. Leaving aside for the moment the intrinsic difficulties of such a position, it was accepted that this would require some degree of educating and informing the population. From Chapter Seven I hope it is clear that even this minimum requirement has not been fulfilled. The efforts to educate in schools, the publicity campaigns at national level and the work of health care teams in the community do not approach the level of comprehensiveness that a consumer led change would require. In other words, agencies of the state have not fulfilled the crucial role that would be necessary for consumer led change to work.

The second compounding factor has been the role of food manufacturers. Their position in the market constrains them to promote their products despite their nutritional properties. This has led to misleading advertising, publicity campaigns, the development of "luxury" high-fat products, sponsorship of "healthy" events (eg. the London Marathon) and a great deal of political pressure for policies which are beneficial to industry, much of which has paid off. The attempts by food manufacturers to defend their products was something given little public consideration by either the state or professionals. Consumer led change, as advocated by the state, does not allow for the political and economic power of food manufacturers who can substantially undermine the best efforts of the Health Education Authority or Primary Health Care Teams. Once again, there appears to be an internal contradiction in the state's position whereby it recognises a public health problem, accepts its validity, but aligns itself with the forces which cause the problem, rather than those which can prevent it.

The third compounding factor, which I would argue is the central problem with the consumer-led philosophy, is the naive perception it has of the demand for food. It conveniently ignores, for example, that the workings of the Common Agricultural Policy can manipulate demand for certain products, and as such, do interfere in the market. But most importantly, it

184

ignores the primary influences over consumer choice and, in particular, it assumes that consumers purchase with perfect knowledge and without financial constraint. Neither of these are necessarily true, not even for the most well informed and the most well-off. The philosophy of consumer led change rests largely on the assumption that there is no price disincentive to make these changes or, in absolute terms, a "healthful" diet is affordable. Again, the relative price of healthful products is higher than its standard counterpart particularly if we take into consideration such things as food availability, taste and cultural preferences. Equally, there is little basis for the assumption that the whole population can afford such products. Yet, this is an area of policy which has been entirely ignored by the state and largely ignored by the food manufacturers. Consequently, there remain strong structural reasons why the consumer led thesis is virtually a non-starter.

It is at this point that comparisons between the experiences of Norway, the United States and Britain become particularly informative. I argued in Chapter Three that the way that diet and heart disease had been tackled in these countries was very much linked to the nature of their political systems and, in particular, the institutional arrangements and division of responsibilities on health between the state and health professionals. In the United States, health professionals have tended to take the lead in suggesting dietary changes, and the role of the state on this issue has reflected its minimalist nature more generally. Equally, given the nature of the state, there are fewer opportunities for state intervention than is the case in Britain. The point is that these divisions of responsibility are known and clear, even if they are disputed. Institutionally, this has meant a diverse health care structure (institution) has emerged which would be inherently more innovative and autonomous. This is consistent with my assertion that health professionals have been the primary force behind dietary change in the United States.

The ideological disposition of the state in Norway is somewhat different; far more interventionist and directive than in the United States. It is not surprising perhaps that it is the state, rather than health professionals, which has taken the lead in developing policies and setting priorities. A state which has historically been interventionist might be expected to respond to professionally defined goals particularly if it has institutionalised relationships which can/will help to implement those policies. In short, the existence of these varying institutional arrangements suggest in themselves where the responsibility and innovativeness may come from.

Britain, of course, falls somewhere in between these two models, although

185

institutionally it has far more in common with Norway. In many ways, this can explain why the consumer-led thesis is inappropriate and why the policies in general are not having the impact on the rates of heart disease that would be expected.

The essence of this argument is simply that the roles of the various interests in this field are not as clearly defined as they might be. It is undoubtedly the case that the British state became more interventionist after WWII and that it has at its disposal structural resources (eg. the NHS) which the United States government does not have. This suggests that in Britain it is the state which would take a lead in advocating dietary change, not professionals. Intuitively, then, it does not seem unreasonable for the state to utilise the resources at its disposal to combat heart disease, but this has not been the position that has been adopted by successive governments. Rather, the state has passed on this responsibility to consumers and health professionals, and so a situation arises in which professional and consumer interests look to the state for guidance, resources and motivation and the state looks straight back at them. Of course, it is the failure of the state to employ the resources that it has, which has been the basis of most of the criticisms of it.

The reason, then, that the roles are not clearly defined is that historically it has been MAFF and the DoH who have controlled policies on diet, food and health. Professional influence and advocacy has been minimal because their sphere of influence has been seen by the state, and themselves, as the NHS. The ideology which generates individual responsibility for primary prevention and consumer led changes in diets, in effect super-imposes the division of responsibilities which are evident in the United States, upon the historical and institutional reality of Britain. Subsequently, neither the state, health professionals or consumers take a lead and the rate of change in heart disease and diets is significantly lower than in either the United States or Norway.

Why Change?

Much the same explanation for policy outcomes will apply to any area of food policy (fibre, sugar, salt, additives, food poisoning, inorganic fertilisers, pesticides, water pollution etc) and to many other areas of primary preventive medicine (lead in petrol, cigarette smoking, road traffic accidents, leukaemia clusters near nuclear installations, health and safety regulations etc). Environmental groups, for example, have suffered from the closed nature of the British decision making process as well. Lowe and Goyder (1983) argue that these groups, which have interests ranging from nuclear power to motorways, are accommodated in peripheral agencies while the upper echelons of central government remain largely inaccessible. In many of these policy areas, we can recognise core interests like those noticeable in MAFF; in the Ministry of Transport are the road hauliers and car manufacturers; in the Department of Energy the electricity generating and supply companies, the UK Atomic Energy Authority (UKAEA), British Nuclear Fuels Ltd (BNFL) etc. In all these cases the semblance of a democratic process is maintained through consultation and collaboration on smaller areas of policy, while larger decisions remain firmly within policy communities. In this respect, then, this case study is not unrepresentative of a common place feature of British policy making.

This, in turn, suggests that such political changes as are necessary, would apply to the broader nature of British policy making.

There is little point in spending a great deal of time discussing the initiatives that would enhance the possibility of a greater reduction in heart disease, because these relate very strongly to the recommendations of health professionals I have already mentioned. There clearly needs to be more inter-departmental coordination; more resources into national campaigns and local community-based programmes; stricter control of the foods offered for sale in terms of compulsory labelling formats and stronger compositional regulations (that is, reducing saturated fat in products); changes to the carcass grading system through fatness and conformation; greater use of the educational facilities in schools and, I would argue, a complete ban on commercial materials used in schools.

These, though, are changes which are specific to the policy area of diet and heart disease, yet, I have consistently argued that this case study demonstrates characteristics of the wider questions on food, health and the political system in general are also problematic.

The political characteristics which have brought us to this point revolve around four key features of decision making in Britain - accessibility; information; integration and accountability. They have consistently militated against public scrutiny of public policy. It is clear that decision making structures within MAFF are inaccessible; they do not voluntarily provide information to interested parties; they are highly integrated, and, as a consequence, there is a distinct lack of accountability in the actions of MAFF. The same sort of argument can be applied to the relationship that exists between MAFF and the DoH.

The problem, therefore, is twofold. In the first place, this type of closed decision making process has prevented consumers judging what is in their own best interests, and hence, policies and policy structures have persisted despite the consequences to public health.

The second problem is that the democratic process is itself undermined. There is no necessary reason why a highly integrated form of decision making should be undemocratic as long as it is accountable, accessible and informative. Problems arise when this is not the case because then the separation of the state and civil society is unclear, and at that point, it can no longer be assumed that the state is acting in the public interest. For policy makers to remain accountable for their actions it is clear that those who wish to scrutinise those actions must know what has been done, and why it has been done. Without this, there is little meaningful way that the processes of public policy formation can be called democratic.

In short, therefore, the decision making process must, I believe, be "opened up" to genuinely incorporate a plurality of opinions. The first step toward this would be to end the anomaly of MAFF having responsibility for promoting the interests of consumers and food and farming interests. This case study has shown that there are occasions when these two responsibilities are contradictory. Either a separate Ministry of Food should be created which would look after consumer interests exclusively, or there should be a new Department of Consumer Affairs which could have a food section within it. These measures would go some way to re-introducing the inter-departmental pluralism which existed in the last war.

This, however, would still leave MAFF with a great deal of control over food policy. Two further measures may help here. Firstly, there should be an end to sponsorship within MAFF, because this institutionalises the relationship between officials and commercial interests. Secondly, some responsibilities should be taken away from MAFF altogether and given to other departments. For example, decisions on research funding should be taken by, or in conjunction with, the DoH, the DES or Consumer Affairs representatives; the advice that MAFF now receives from the Food Advisory Committee or its own Scientific Division should come from, or be supplemented by, a sub-central agency without allegiance to MAFF itself. All these measures would help to avoid the recurrent problem that MAFF is all too often judge and jury of its own case.

Similar measures should be applied to the DoH as well. Certainly, in terms of the controls that the DoH can exercise over the advice it receives from its advisory committees there is room for improvement. This could take the form of, for example, strengthening the role of the Health Education Authority so that it, too, can instigate a COMA panel to advise in certain areas of policy. Equally, there could be an extension of the role of the National Audit Office, or the creation of a monitoring bureau which would assess policies like those for diet and heart disease not only in terms of their cost-effectiveness, but also in terms of whether the policies bear any resemblance to the political undertakings upon which they are based.

Finally, to facilitate the provision of information and the accessibility of decision making structures there must be (1) freedom of information, by which I mean that restrictive rules on the disclosure of information should be avoided, and some compulsory disclosures should be necessary in terms of both justifications for policy decisions and explanations of policy processes (who said what to whom etc.); (2), there must be a formalisation of the political relationships within MAFF, rather than the ad hoc consultation process, and these new arrangements should institutionalise a role for health and consumer interests. This would probably take the form of standing committees on, for example, food labelling, composition etc.

Of course, there can be many objections to these suggestions on the basis of, for example, the practicality of decision making by committee or, indeed, the legitimacy of it given that the electoral process is supposed to provide the major democratic element of the political system. My argument rests primarily upon the belief that not only does the present system not work, in the sense that it does not operate for the public good, but that it is democratically undesirable. I do not doubt that the suggestions I have given may well replace one set of problems with another in some instances, but it seems to me that if nothing else, they illustrate what is wrong with the system as it stands at the moment and as such, are useful.

Policy Futures?

The future of policies which are related to diet and health is difficult to predict with any certainty. My own view is that the food supply, that is, manufactured food, will continue to be reformed gradually by MAFF but in ways which can be easily absorbed by industry. So, it is perfectly possible that the list of additives used in food will be reduced, indeed it has been, but this reduction will not necessarily correlate to the most dangerous additives, only those which are dispensable to industry. Similarly, the rate of CHD will continue to fall, but that it will remain inversely related to class and that this relation will, in fact, strengthen, that is, a higher proportion of cases will fall in the lower socio-economic groups. We can expect an expansion of organic farming and more low fat products on super-market shelves, primarily because both can command premium prices. Again, this is comforting inasmuch as these are desirable but do not, in themselves, constitute a comprehensive response to the problems inherent in the food supply. It is not possible, even as a short term solution, to solve the whole problem of food by adding to the volume of food available; the problem is qualitative as much as quantitative.

In the short to medium term there is little evidence to suggest that comprehensive, preventive, community based solutions will be forthcoming. The NHS reforms which are now under discussion give conflicting signs for the future, largely because they are not intended to promote preventive medicine. On the one hand GP's are encouraged to perform rudimentary preventive practice such as establishing height\weight ratios and taking blood pressure. On the other hand, they are working to budgets which encourage them to expand their patient lists and reduce the time available to each patient in consultation. These somewhat contradictory indicators are not unusual within the confines of this case study, and demonstrate the difficulties of establishing any firm commitment on the part of the state to "a" nutrition policy or "a" policy on prevention. There is nothing within the neo-liberal philosophy of the "commodification of everything" which lends itself to preventing disease; it is primarily a scheme to reduce costs within curative systems. As such, it tends toward reinforcing the view that medicine should be practised within a discrete health care system which has to operate with its own internal market. My argument has been that, in fact, this is not the way health care must go in the future; rather, it is the fact that medicine is too discrete and is not more fully integrated into other societal structures which causes many of the health problems of western societies.

The political costs to any government of changing their role with regard to food are almost inevitably going to be; short term price inflation; the disaffection of industry; an increase in public expenditure and some degree of consumer confusion. These costs are unlikely to be incurred lightly. Even if they were, if price inflation is likely, then the policy of, for example, requiring unnecessary saturated fat to be removed from products, will only succeed if consumers have the ability to pay for these products. Invariably, economic imperatives have established themselves as norms which are too costly or too prized to challenge.

On this scenario, which appears to be the most likely one, we shall not see the formulation of anything approaching a comprehensive policy. Rather, a regular series of reassuring initiatives will be announced which are partial contributions to changing the British diet.

Politically, the method of decision making will remain largely the same. MAFF and the DoH have been in public conflict over food poisoning but this is unlikely to be repeated in other areas of food policy simply because of the political embarrassment that such disagreements cause incumbent governments. There does not appear to be any shift of power resources away from MAFF, nor any change in the role of the DoH. As such, one must assume that while the division of responsibilities between the two departments remains the same and, while access to MAFF is restricted, then the policy communities and networks will continue to make policy largely as before. Indeed, Lowe and Goyder found that MAFF was one of the most inaccessible central departments of all, and there is little evidence to suggest that this has changed (1983;p63-65).

There are perhaps two factors which could substantially alter this scenario. This first is the partial greening of British politics. There are a number of social forces which are pushing for changes in the food supply; one of the more prominent of these is currently the green movement. What is particularly interesting is the fact that environmental issues exist as problems primarily because of the effects of industrialisation, in much the same way as I have argued that the problems of the food supply do. The solution to many of these problems, from whaling and the fur trade to acid rain and the green house effect, all require the acknowledgement by governments and publics that (1) markets and industrialisation need to be managed and controlled and (2) the effects of industrialisation can be total and indiscriminate. Issues such as pesticide residues and the pollution of the water supply have already established the connection between environmental issues and consumption and also that environmental issues are often health issues.

My argument is, therefore, that an acknowledgement within political structural elites that broader political controls over industrial and agricultural processes are necessary for long-term security may extend to those processes which supply our food. I have argued all along that it is the autonomy of the market and the states relationship to it that has constrained changes in the British food supply. The advent of environmental problems may re-define that relationship and, by doing so, establish new norms of state intervention on public health grounds.

A second variable which may affect the nature of the British food supply is the increasing integration of the European Community. The extent to which this may lead to changes has been qualified by the inability of member states to agree on compositional standards for certain products, hence the problems of British chocolate not qualifying as a chocolate by

European standards because of its cocoa content. There have been similar problems with German sausages, for example. Consequently, it has been agreed that what is allowed in one country must be allowed in others for the purposes of export and import and this does, of course, curtail the likely changes in British compositional standards. Nevertheless, as a qualification to the apparently predictable pattern of British food policy, the role of the EC cannot be excluded, after all, it has already had some impact in terms of the declaration of additives (E numbers). Equally, the West German ban on British beef imports because of BSE (mad cow disease) is an example of how greater economic inter-dependence may encourage reforms where the domestic repercussions of policies could not.

Future Research

Research into the effect of the Single European Act on the nature of the British food supply would be extremely worthwhile and would help to establish the extent to which MAFF can expect to retain control over the nature of the food supply in the future.

There are a number of other areas for future research which could both extend the analysis presented here and provide useful comparative material. There are, for example, very few case studies which relate to issues in preventive medicine. It would be very interesting to know whether, and to what extent, the characteristics of this policy area hold true in other areas. In particular, it would be useful to know the political differences between primary prevention that is administered within the NHS and prevention which is applied, for example, in the workplace. Is it the case, for example, that preventive health measures are always constrained by economic considerations, or do certain institutional arrangements (policy communities, for example) coincide with a reduction in health considerations in public policy?

There is certainly a place for more up-to-date quantitative research into the effects of price on consumer purchases of healthful products, the availability of these products and a review of these in relation to Income Support levels. If, as present research suggests, there is a strong correlation between price, income and consumption, this would almost certainly have been strengthened within the past five years or so.

Given that the state has accepted some degree of responsibility for the vulnerable sections of the population, the re-definition by the present government of who are vulnerable (targeted as opposed to universal benefits) presents an opportunity to establish the effect that this re-definition has had on the nutritional well-being of the population.

In terms of food policy, topics for further research are also plentiful. I have contended that I believe that the explanations I have given for policies on diet and heart disease would also apply to other policy areas within MAFF. Nevertheless, an academic, as opposed to a journalistic, study of food additives, agro-chemicals, and the very powerful sugar industry, would provide invaluable comparative material.

*   *   *   *   *

The problems of a late twentieth century industrialised society are unique because of the capacity of these societies to affect everyone. It is no longer possible to isolate particular groups from others beyond the fact that social class is invariably inversely related to the worst effects of these societies. This capacity challenges not only the British government, but others, to reassess the costs they believe their populations should incur for the sake of the maintenance of their economic priorities.

The case of diet and CHD is important in its own right because it is a major health problem across national boundaries. But it also highlights many political and economic problems which exist in the food supply and in areas of preventive medicine generally. In essence, it touches on the question of the quality of life and how it is defined politically. Such a definition, which exists at the level of volumes and quantities, is unsustainable in the long term and, in the interests of public health, needs to be redefined.

Bibliography

ACARD (Advisory Council for Applied Research and Development), (1982), *The Food Industry and Technology,* HMSO:London.

Acheson, Sir E.D. (1986), "Food Policy, Nutrition and the Government",*in*, Proceedings of the Nutrition Society, 45, p131-138.

Acheson, R.M. (1988), "Prevention versus Cure:Use of Resources in the National Health Service", *in,* Keynes, M., Coleman, D.A. and Dimsdale, N.H., *The Political Economy of Health and Welfare,* Macmillan in Association with the Eugenics Society:London.

Aldcroft, D.H. (1983), *The British Economy Between the Wars,* Philip Allen:Oxford.

Alford, R.A. (1975), *Health Care Politics,* University of Chicago Press:Chicago.

Allsop, J. (1984), *Health Policy and the National Health Service,* Longman:London.

Allsop, J. (1989), "Health", *in,* McCarthy, M., *The New Politics of*

Welfare:An Agenda for the 1990's?, Macmillan:London.

Ball, K. P., and Turner, R., Letter, British Medical Journal, 7th Aug 1976.

Ball, K. P., and Turner. R., Letter, British Medical Journal, 21st Sept 1984.

Bartley, M. (1985), "Coronary Heart Disease and the Public Health", *Sociology of Health and Illness*, Vol.7, November, p289-313.

BBC, (1986), "O'Donnell Investigates", April.

The BCCCA (Biscuit, Cake, Chocolate and Confectionary Alliance), (1987), Letter from the President to the Minister of Agriculture, Mr. Jopling.

Bell, D., (1976), *The Coming of Post-Industrial Society*, Peregrine Books:Harmondsworth.

Benson, J. K. (1982), "Networks and Policy Sectors:A Framework for Extending Interorganisational Analysis." *in* Rogers, D. and Whitten, D. (eds), *Interorganisational Coordination*, Iowa State University Press:Ames, Iowa.

Benton, T. (1984), *The Rise and Fall of Structural Marxism: Althusser and his Influence*, Macmillan:London.

Beveridge, W.H. (1928), *British Food Control*, Oxford University Press:London.

Black, N. (et al), (1984), *Health and Disease:A Reader*, Open University Press:Glasgow.

Blythe, C. (1976), "Eating Our Way Out Of Debt and Disease." New Scientist, Vol.70, p278-80.

BMRB (British Market Research Bureau Ltd), (1985), *Consumer Attitudes to and Understanding of Nutrition Labelling: Quantitative Stage*, BMRB: London.

Boyd-Orr, J. (1936), *Food Health and Income*, Macmillan:London.

Boyd-Orr, J. (1940), *Nutrition in War*, Fabian Society Tract Series No. 257:London.

Brand, J.A. (1971), "The Politics of Fluoridation:A Community Conflict", *Political Studies* XIX No.4, p430-439.

British Medical Association, (1986), *Diet, Nutrition and Health*, BMA:London.

British Medical Journal, Leader, Sept', 1972.

British Medical Journal, July 6th 1974.

British Medical Journal,1976, p881-882.

British Medical Journal, Leader, No.6444 p509-510.

British Medical Journal, 1987.

BSSRS (British Society for Social Responsibility in Science) (1986), New Food Politics Conference, London, November.

Burnett, J. (1979), *Plenty and Want*, Scholar Press:London.

Cannon, G. (1984), The Times, June 11th, p13.

Cannon, G. (1987), *The Politics of Food*, Century: London.

Cannon, G. (1987b), *Universal Agreement on Food and Health*, Unpublished.

Carnoy, M. (1984), *The State and Political Theory*, Princeton University Press:Princeton.

CECG (Consumers in the European Community Group), (1984), "Enough is Enough: The Common Agricultural Policy", CECG: London.

CECG (1985), "The Common Agricultural Policy and Diet", CECG: London.

CECG, (1987), Comments by Consumers in the European Community Group (CECG) on the European Oils and Fats Regime, London.

Channel 4, (1984), "Food for Thought", in association with the HEC.

Cohen, G.A. (1978), *Karl Marx's Theory of History: A Defence*, Clarendon Press:Oxford.

Coller, F.H. (1925), *A State Trading Adventure*, Oxford University Press:London.

Committee of Public Accounts, (1986), *Preventive Medicine*, HMSO:London.

Consumers Association (1986), "Nutrition Labelling-One Step to Better Information-But Not Enough", Press Release.

CPG (Coronary Prevention Group) (1986), *Farming, Food and the Prevention of Coronary Heart Disease,* Proceedings of a Conference held on 1 December 1986, CPG: London.

Dalzell, I. (1985), Letter to MAFF on the Fat Content Labelling of Food -

NFU response.

Darke, S.J. (1979), "A Nutrition Policy for Britain", Journal of Human Nutrition, Vol.33, p438-444.

Darling,G. (1941), *The Politics of Food*, The Labour Book Service:London.

Davies, C. (1984), "General Practice and the Pull of Prevention", *Sociology of Health and Illness*, Vol.6, No.3, p267-289.

DoH. (1989), *Working for Patients*, HMSO:London.

DHSS, (1974), *Diet and Coronary Heart Disease*, Report of a Panel of the Committee on the Medical Aspects of Food Policy, HMSO:London.

DHSS, (1976), *Priorities for the Health and Social Services in England*, HMSO:London.

DHSS, (1976), *Prevention and Health:Everybodies Business*, HMSO:London.

DHSS, (1977), *Prevention and Health*, Cmd. 7047. HMSO:London.

DHSS, (1979), *Prevention and Health: Eating for Health*, HMSO:London.

DHSS, (1981), *Prevention and Health: Avoiding Heart Attacks*, HMSO:London.

DHSS, (1983), *NHS Management Inquiry Report*, HMSO:London.

DHSS, (1984), *Diet and Cardiovascular Disease*, Committee on the Medical Aspects of Food Policy, HMSO:London.

DHSS, (1987), *Promoting Better Health: The Governments Programme for Improving Primary Health Care*, Cmd. 249, HMSO:London.

DHSS, (1988), *Working for Patients*, Cm.555, HMSO:London.

DHSS, (1988), *Public Health in England*, Cmd. 289, HMSO:London.

Doll, Sir R.(1983), British Medical Journal, Vol.286, p448.

Doyal, L. and Epstein, S.S. (1983), *Cancer in Britain:The Politics of Prevention*, Pluto:Bristol.

Drummond, J. C. and Wilbraham, A. (1964), *The Englishman's Food*, Jonathan Cape:London.

Dubos, R. (1960), *Mirage of Health*, Allen and Unwin:London, *quoted in*, Wistow, G. (1989), "The Health Service Policy Community:Professionals Pre-Emminent or Under Challenge?, Paper to the Policy Networks Conference, University of Essex, June 30-July 1.

Dunleavy, P., (1982), "Quasi-Governmental Sector Professionalism." *in* Barker, A. (ed) *Quango's in Britain*, Macmillan:London.

Dunleavy, P., (1981), "Professions and Policy Change." *Public Administration Bulletin* No.36 August.

Elliot, Mr. (1934), Parliamentary Debates Commons, Vol.286 19th Feb-9th March Col. 503-4.

Ennals, Lord. (1984), Hansard, House of Lords, Vol. 455, 25th July, p381.

Ennals, Lord. (1986), Speech to the Institute of Health Food Retailing, *quoted in*, Cannon, G. (1987), *The Politics of Food*, Century:London.

Earl of Caithness, (1986), Hansard, House of Lords, Vol. 455, 25th July.

Etzioni-Halevy, E. (1985), *The Knowledge Elite and the Failure of Prophecy*, George, Allen and Unwin Ltd:London.

European Commission (1979), "Council Directive (79/112/EEC) on the approximation of the laws of the Member States to the labelling, presentation and advertising of foodstu: s for sale to the ultimate consumer". *Official Journal of the European Communities*, No. L 33.

European Commission (1985), "Commission Regulation (EEC) No. 1716/85....on laying down detailed rules for the supply of milk and certain milk products to schoolchildren", *Official Journal of the European Communities*, No. L 165/6.

Farchi, I. (1984), "Multi-Factoral Primary Prevention Trials of Coronary Heart Disease." *Revue D'Epidemilogic et de Sante Publique*, Vol.32: No. 3-4, p219-224.

Farrent, W. and Russell, J, (1985), *The Politics of Health Information*, Bedford Way Papers 28, Institute of Education, University of London.

Feedback, (1987), The Trade Paper of the Food and Drink Federation, November Issue.

Feedback, (1987), No.20 August Issue, Page 1.

FDF (Food and Drink Federation) (undated), "Common Sense About Food", FDF Publicity Leaflet.

FDF (Food and Drink Federation) (1987), "FDF Slams European Commission Oils and Fats Tax Proposal", FDF News.

The Financial Times,(1988), 20th October.

The Food Programme (1989), BBC Radio 4, 6th March, 7.20pm.

Fletcher, D. (1986), "Row over teenage diet report", Daily Telegraph, 3rd April.

FSC (Food Standards Committee), (1980), *Meat Products*, HMSO:London.

Freckleton, A. (1985), "Who is Shaping the Nutritional Label?", Food Policy Research, University of Bradford.

Freidson, E. (1970), *Professional Dominance: The Social Construction of Medical Care*, Aldine:Chicago.

French, C. (1986), "The Farmers Response", *in, Farming, Food and the Prevention of Coronary Heart Disease*, Proceedings of a Conference, Coronary Prevention Group: London.

Gamble, A. (1986), *Britain in Decline*, Macmillan:London.

Giddens, A. (1978), *Central Problems in Social Theory*, Macmillan:London.

Gowes, A. and Dawney, I, (1986), "Another Shot of Politics for the Beef Farmers", Financial Times, 24th January.

Grant, W. (1983), *The UK Food Processing Industry*, International Institute of Management:Berlin.

Grant, W.P., Paterson, W. and Whitson, C. (1988), *Government and the Chemical Industry*, Oxford University Press:London.

Gray, P.S, (1986), "What Role can the EEC Play in Encouraging Farmers to Respond to Current Dietary Recommendations?", Paper from, The Head of Foodstuffs Division, Commission of the European Community

Gray, A. and Jenkins, W.I. (1985), *Administrative Politics in British Government*, Wheatsheaf:Brighton.

Griffiths, R. (1988), *Community Care:Agenda for Action*, HMSO:London.

Gillie, O. (1985), "Guide to Healthy Eating Blocked", Sunday Times, 4th August.

Gutzwiller, F., Martin, J., Lehmann, P. (1987) "Primary Prevention of Cardiovascular Disease in Switzerland." World Health Forum, Vol.8.

Ham, C. (1981), *Policy Making in the NHS*, Macmillan:London.

Ham, C. (1986), *Managing Health Services*, SAUS:Bristol.

Ham, C. and Hill, M. (1984), *The Policy Process in the Modern Capitalist State*, Wheatsheaf Harvester:London.

Hammond,R.J. (1951), *Food Volume One: The Growth of Policy*, HMSO and Longmans:London.

Hansard (1984), Vol.64 c147-154.

Hardman, R.J. (1981), "The British Food Processing Industry", Jordan and Sons (Surveys) Ltd:London

Harrington, G. (1985), "Meat in the Modern World: The Eighth Lawson Lecture", Meat and Livestock Commission: London.

Harrison, S. (1988), *Managing the National Health Service*, Chapman and Hall:London.

Harrison, A. and Gretton, J. (1987), *Health Care UK 1987:An Economic, Social and Political Audit*, Policy Journals:Bristol.

Harrison, S., Hunter, D., Marnock, G. and Pollitt, C. (1989), *The Impact of General Management in the National Health Service*, Nuffield Institute for Health Services Studies and the Open University, *quoted in*, Wistow, G. (1989), "The Health Services Policy Community: Professionals Pre-Emminent or Under Challenge?", Paper to the Policy Networks Conference, University of Essex, June 30-July 1.

Haywood, S. and Alaszewski, A. (1980), *Crisis in the Health Service*, Croom Helm:London.

Haywood, S. and Hunter, D.J. (1982), "Consultative Processes in Health Policy in the United Kingdom: A View from the Centre." *Public Administration*, Vol.60 p143-62.

Health Education Authority, (1989), *Strategic Plan 1990-95*, HEA:London.

Health Education Council, (1983), *Report of an Ad-Hoc Working Party of the National Advisory Committee on Nutrition Education (NACNE)*, HEC:London.

Health Education Council, (1985), "Eating for a Healthier Heart-The JACNE Leaflet", HEC:London.

Health Education Council, (1986), "Guide to Healthy Eating", HEC: London.

Heclo, H. (1978), "Issue Networks and the Executive Establishment." *in*, A. King (eds), *The New American Political System*, American Enterprise Inc.: Washington D.C. p87-124.

Held, D. (1989), *Models of Democracy*, Polity Press:Oxford.

HMSO, (1928), The Registrar Generals Statistical Review of England and Wales for the Year 1928.

HMSO, (1954), The Registrar Generals Statistical Review of England and Wales for the Year 1951.

Hogwood, B.W. and Gunn, L.A., (1984), *Policy Analysis for the Real World*, Oxford University Press:Oxford.

Holderness, B.A. (1985), *British Agriculture Since 1945*, Manchester University Press:Manchester.

Hollingham, M.A. and Howarth, R.W. (1989), *British Milk Marketing and the Common Agricultural Policy:The Origins of Confusion and Crisis*, Avebury, in Association with the Adam Smith Institute:Aldershot.

Hollingsworth, D., (1985), "Rationing and Economic Constraint on Food Consumption in Britain Since the Second World War." *in* Oddy, D.J. and Miller, D.S., *Diet and Health in Modern Britain*, Croom Helm:London.

Hollingsworth, J.R. (1986), *A Political Economy of Medicine*, John Hopkins University Press:London.

Honigsbaum, F., (1970), *The Struggle for the Ministry of Health:1914-1919*, Occasional Papers in Social Administration No.37, G.Bell and Sons:London.

Howarth, R.W. (1985), *Farming for Farmers? A Critique of Agricultural Support Policy*, Institute of Economic Affairs:London.

Hunter, D.J. (1980), *Coping With Uncertainty*, Wiley:London.

Illich, I. (1976), *Limits to Medicine- Medical Nemisis:The Expropriation of Health*, Penguin:Harmondsworth.

Illsley, R., (1980), *Professional or Public Health?*, Nuffield:Oxford.

Ingham, G. (1984), *Capitalism Divided: The City and Industry in British Social Development*, Macmillan:London.

Interdepartmental Committee on Physical Deterioration, (1904) Cmd. 2175.

Interdisciplinary Workshop Conference-Canterbury, (1984), *Coronary Heart Disease: Plans for Action*, Pitman:London.

James, P. (1989), "What COMA Set Out to Acheive", *in*, Royal Society of Medicine, *Dietary Fat and Heart Disease:Progress Since COMA?*, Round Table Series No. 13. Royal Society of Medicine Services:London.

Johnson, T.J., (1972), *Professions and Power*, MacMillan:London.

Jones, A (undated), "Recommended Changes in the Human Diet: The Impact on Agricultural Policy, Synopsis of a Paper, Rowett Research Institute, Aberdeen.

Jones, A. (1986), "How Farmers can Influence the Composition of Farm Products", *in*, *Farming, Food and the Prevention of Coronary Heart Disease*, Proceedings of a Conference, Coronary Prevention Group: London.

Jordan, A.G., (1981), "Iron Triangles, Wooley Corporatism and Elastic Nets", *Journal of Public Policy* Vol.1 No.1.

Journal of the Royal College of Physicians of London, Vol.35 No.276, p59-60.

Jupe, G. (1985), "Food Policy Issues and Government Regulations, Paper to the Food Policy Issues and the Food Industries Conference, University of Reading, 12-13 September.

Laffin,M. (1986), *Professionalism and Policy*, Gower:Aldershot.

Klein, R. (1983), *The Politics of the NHS*, Longman:London.

The Lancet, 25th March 1933.

The Lancet, 19th May 1934.

The Lancet, 21st March 1936.

The Lancet, 13th April 1940.

The Lancet, March 14th 1942.

The Lancet, 3rd October 1942.

The Lancet Leader, 1983,p601-602.

The Lancet, 1987, p601-602.

Landsborough-Thomson, A. (1975), *Half a Century of Medical Research Volume Two*, HMSO:London.

Lang, T., Andrews, H., Bedale, C., Hannon, E. (1984), *Jam Tomorrow?*, Food Policy Unit: Manchester Polytechnic.

Lang,T. (1986), Address to the New Food Politics Conference of the British Society for Social Responsibility in Science, Nov'1986: London.

Lee, P. R. (1979), "Do We Need a Federal Department of Health?", *in*, D. Cater, and P.R. Lee, *Politics of Health*, Robert. E. Kreiger Publishing Co: New York.

Lindblom, Charles, E. (1977), *Politics and Markets: The World's Political-Economic Systems*, Basic Books:New York.

Lloyd, E.M.H. (1924), *Experiments in State Control*, Oxford University Press:London.

Lowe, P. and Goyder, J. (1983), *Environmental Groups in Politics*, George, Allen and Unwin:London.

Luba,A, and Cole-Hamilton, I, (1986), *Food labelling: A Critique of the Governments Proposed Fat Content Labelling Regulations and Nutritional Labelling Guidelines*, London Food Commission Briefing Paper: London.

Lukes, S. (1978), *Essays in Social Theory*, Macmillan:London.

Lukes. S. (1984), *Power:A Radical View*, Macmillan:London.

MAFF (1978), *The Manual of Nutrition*, HMSO:London.

MAFF (1984), *The Meat Products and Spreadable Fish Products Regulations*, Statutory Instruments: Food Composition and Labelling. HMSO:London.

MAFF (1985), "Government Proposals on the COMA Report: Food-Fat Content and Nutritional Labelling", Press Release.

MAFF (1986a), *Proposals for Fat Content of Food (Labelling) Regulations*, MAFF:London.

MAFF (1986b), *Revised Draft MAFF Guidelines on Nutrition Labelling*, Standards division, MAFF: London.

Marsh, D. (1988), "The Marxist Theory of the State", mimeo, Department of Government, University of Essex.

MSMA (Margarine and Shortening Manufacturers Association) (1987), Press Release on Oils and Fats Tax.

Mason, T.J.R. (1985), "A Food Retailer View of Food Policy Issues", Paper to the Food Policy Issues and the Food Industries Conference, University of Reading, 12-13 September.

Massey, A., (1985)"Professional Elites and the BNFL", *Politics* Vol.6 No.1.

MLC (Meat and Livestock Commission), (1986), "Producing Lean Meat", Leaflet.

McKeown, T. (1976), *The Role of Medicine:Dream, Mirage or Nemisis?*, Nuffield:Oxford.

McLachlan, G. (1973), *Portfolio for Health 2*, Nuffield Provincial Hospital Trust:Oxford.

McNair, A. (1982), "Screening for IHD is Effective.", *General Practitioner*, 22nd Feb' 1988.

MRC, (Medical Research Council),(1937), *Annual report, quoted in*, Landsborough-Thomson, A. (1975), *Half a Century of Medical Research*, HMSO:London.

Miliband, R. (1976), *The State in Capitalist Society*, Quartet:London

Ministry of Health, (1944), *A National Health Service*, Cmd. 6502, HMSO:London, *quoted in*, Wistow, G. (1989), "The Health Service Policy Community:Professionals Pre-Eminent or Under Challenge? Paper to the Policy Networks Conference, University of Essex, June 30-July 1.

Ministry of Health (1964), *On the State of the Public Health*, HMSO:London.

MMC (Monopolies and Mergers Commission), (1981), *Discounts to Retailers*, HC 311, HMSO:London.

Montague, S. (1985), *Healthy Eating and the NHS*, Food Policy Research, University of Bradford.

Morris, J.N. (1951), "Recent History of Coronary Heart Disease I and II", The Lancet,i, p1-7 andp 69-73.

The Multiple Risk Factor Intervention Trial (MRFIT), (1981), "The Methods and Impact of Intervention Over Four Years", Preventive Medicine Vol.10:p387.

Murray, K.A.H., (1955), *Agriculture*, HMSO and Longmans:London.

NAO (National Audit Office), (1989), *National Health Service: Coronary Heart Disease*, HMSO: London.

National Consumer Council, (1986), "Response by the National Consumer Council to the Governments Proposals on Nutritional Labelling", NNC: London.

National Forum for Coronary Heart Disease Prevention, (1988), *Coronary Heart Disease Prevention: Action in the UK 1984-1987*, Health Education Authority:London.

Navarro, V. (1976), "The Mode of State Intervention in the Health Sector", *in*, Black, N. (ed), *Health and Disease:A Reader*, Open University Press:Glasgow. First published in, Navarro, V., *Medicine Under Capitalism*, Prodist:New York.

NEDC (National Economic Development Committee), (1986), *Review of the Food and Drink Manufacturing Industry*, NEDO:London.

The New England Journal of Medicine, Leader, Vol. 312, No.16 1985, pp1053-1055.

Nursing Times, Vol.83, No.15, pp24-26.

OFT (Office of Fair Trading), (1985), *Competition and Retailing*, HMSO:London.

Office of Health Economics, (1982), *Coronary Heart Disease: The Scope for Prevention*, The Office of Health Economics:Luton.

Office of Health Economics, (1985), *Measurement of Health*, OHE:Luton.

Olsen, J. P. (1983), *Organised Democracy:Political Institutions in a Welfare State-The Case of Norway*, Universitetsforlarget:Oslo.

Owen, D. (1977), *In Sickness and in Health*, Quartet:London.

Patten, J. (1984), Written reply to M.Shersby, Hansard, Vol.45.

Personal Correspondence (A), Interview with Health Education Official, 1987.

Personal Correspondence (B), Interview with MAFF Official, 1986.

Personal Correspondence (C), Interview with Journalist, 1988.

Personal Correspondence (D), Interview with Member of the COMA Panel, 1986.

Personal Correspondence (E), Letter from J. Michael Shersby MP, 1986.

Personal Correspondence (F), Interview with MAFF Official, 1986.

Personal Correspondence (G), Interview with Representative of the Dairy Industry, 1986.

Personal Correspondence (H), Interview with Representative of the Meat Industry, 1986.

Personal Correspondence (J), Interview with Health Education Authority Officials, 1988.

Personal Correspondence (K), Interview with Representative of the Meat Industry, 1987.

Personal Correspondence (L), Interview with Representative of European Consumers, 1987.

Personal Correspondence (M), Interview with the Director of the Coronary Prevention Group (Anne Dillon), 1987.

Personal Correspondence (N), Telephone Conversation with a Representative of the BMA; 1988.

Personal Correspondence (0), Interview with DHSS official, 1986.

Personal Correspondence (P), Interview with Retailing Executive, 1987.

Personal Correspondence (Q), Interview with Consumer Representative, 1986).

Pollard, S. (1983), *The Development of the British Economy*, Arnold:London.

Preventive Medicine, Vol.14, No.3 1985, p279-292.

Puska, P. et al, (1981), *The North Karelia Project: Evaluation of a Comprehensive Community Programme for Control of Cardiovascular Disease in North Karelia Finland 1972-1977,* Copenhagen: Regional Office for Europe WHO.

Pyke, M, (1952), *The Townsman's Food*, Turnstile Press:London.

Pyke, M, (1985), "The Impact of Modern Food Technology on Nutrition in the Twentieth Century," *in*, Oddy, D. J, and Miller, D.S. *Diet and Health in Modern Britain*, Croom Helm:London.

Rayner, M. (1989), "The Truth about the British Diet", *New Scientist* Vol.123, No. 1674, p44-48.

Read, M.D. (1989), "Networks of the Tobacco Industry:A Strategy for Defence", Paper to the Policy Networks Conference, University of Essex, June 30-July 1.

Rhodes, R.A.W.,(1985), "Power Dependence, Policy Commmunities and Inter-Governmental Networks." Paper to PAC Conference.

Rhodes, R.A.W. (1986), *The National World of Local Government,* Allen and Unwin:London.

Rhodes, R.A.W. and Marsh, D. (1991), *Policy Communities in British Politics,* Oxford University Press:London. Forthcoming.

Richardson, J.J., and Jordan, A.G., (1979), *Governing Under Pressure*, Robertson:Oxford.

Ringen, K. (1977), "The Norwegian Food and Nutrition Policy", *American Journal of Public Health*, Vol.67, No.6 p550-551

Ringen, K. (1979), "The "New Ferment" in National Health Policies: The Case of Norway's Nutrition and Food Policy." *Social Science and Medicine*, Vol. 13C, p33-41.

Ringen, K. (1983), "Norway's Nutrition and Food Policy" in McClaren, D.S. (ed), *Nutrition in the Community*, John Wiley and Sons Ltd:London .

Robbins, C. and Bowman, J. (1983), "Nutrition and Agriculture Policy in the United Kingdom." in, McClaren, D.S. (ed), *Nutrition in the Community*, John Wiley and Sons Ltd:London.

Rose, G., Reid, D.D., Hamilton, P. J. S., McCartney, P., Keen, H., Jarrett, R. J., (1977), "Myocardial Ischaemia, risk factors and death from coronary heart disease", Lancet (i), p105-109.

The Royal College of General Practitioners (1981), *Prevention of Arterial Disease in General Practice*, Report from General Practice Number 19.

The Royal College of General Practitioners (1981a), *Health and Prevention in General Practice*, Report from General Practice Number 18.

The Royal College of Physicians of London and the British Cardiac Society-Report of a Joint Working Party, (1976), "The Prevention of Coronary Heart Disease." *Journal of the Royal College of Physicians*. Vol.10, No.3 April 1976.

Royal Commission, (1905), *Report on the Supply of Food and Raw Materials in Wartime*, Cmd. 2643.

Royal Norwegian Ministry of Health and Social Affairs, (1981-2), *On the Follow-Up of the Norwegian Nutrition Policy*, Report to the Storting No.11.

Royal Society, (1916), Report of the Physiological (War) Committee, Cmd.8421.

Royal Society of Medicine Services, (1989), *Dietary Fat and Heart Disease: Progress Since COMA?*, Royal Society of Medicine Services; Oxford

Runciman, (1916), Hansard, 86 HC Deb 55 488 col.

Saunders, P., (1984), *We Can't Afford Democracy Too Much*, University of Sussex.

SCOPA (Seed Crushers and Oil Processors Association) (1987), "SCOPA Stresses Opposition to Oils and Fats Tax Proposals", Press Release

Scott, A. (1987), "EEC Plans Food Gift for the Poor", The Guardian, 21st January.

Self, P. and Storing, H.J. (1962), *The State and the Farmer*, George Allen and Unwin Ltd:London.

Senate Select Committee, (1977), *On Nutrition and Human Needs*, US Senate:Washington.

Shaper, G. (1989), "COMA recommendations and the British Regional

Heart Study." *in*, The Royal Society of Medicine Services, *Dietary Fat and Heart Disease: Progress Since COMA?*, Royal Society of Medicine Services:Oxford.

Sharp, L.J., (1985), "Central Coordination and the Policy Network." Political Studies Vol.XXXIII No.3, Sept'.

Shrimpton, D. (1985) *on*, World in Action "The Great Food Scandal", *quoted in*, Cannon, G (1987), *The Politics of Food*, Century :London.

Skocpol, T. (1984), "Bringing the State Back In: Strategies of Analysis in Current Research.", *in*, Evans, P. (et al), *Bringing the State Back In*, Cambridge University Press:Cambridge.

Skuse, A. (1976), *Government Intervention and Industrial Policy*, Heinemann:London.

Smith, A. and Jacobson, B. (eds) (1988), *The Nation's Health*, King's Fund:London.

Smith, M.J. (1988), "Undermining a Closed Policy Community? The Case of Agriculture", Essex Papers in Politics and Government, No.51.

Smith, M.J. (1989), "The Annual Price Review:The Emergence of a Corporatist Institution?" Political Studies, Vol:XXXVII, p81-96.

Smith, M.J. (1990), "Pluralism, Reformed Pluralism and Neopluralism:the Role of Pressure Groups in Policy-Making." *Political Studies*, XXXVIII, p302-322.

Span, R.N. (1940), "The Use of Advisory Bodies in the Ministry of Health." *in* Vernon, R.V. and Mansergh, N. (eds) *Advisory Bodies*, G. Allen and Unwin Ltd:London.

Starling, E.H., (1919), *The Feeding of Nations*, Longmans, Green and Co.:London.

Street, J. (1988), "Policy Advice on AIDS", Paper to the ECPR Joint Workshop on Policy Advice to Government, Rimini, 10-15 April.

Stones, R. (1988), "What's Right and What's Wrong With Vogel's Pluralist Critique of Lindblom: And What Would Be Better." Essex Paper in Politics and Government, No. 57. Dep't of Gov't: University of Essex.

Stones, R. (1988b), "State-Finance Relations in Britain: A De-Centred Approach", Paper to the ECPR Joint Session of Workshops, Rimini, Italy.

Sunday Times (1983), "Censored-A Diet for Life and Death", 11th July.

Susie Fisher Research, (1985), *Consumer Attitudes to and Understanding of Nutrition Labelling: Qualitative Stage*, Susie Fisher Research: London.

Swinbank, A., Burns, J.A. and Beard, N.F., (1985), "Economic Aspects of Food Policy Issues", University of Reading, Department of Agricultural Economics and Management:Discussion Paper No. 85/1.

Tait, I. (1985), "The Primary Health Care Team", *in*, Telling-Smith, G. (ed), *Health Education and General Practice*, OHE:Luton.

Telling-Smith, G. (ed) (1985), *Health Education and General Practice*, OHE:London

The Times, (1986), Anon, "Children's Snack Diet Criticised", 4th April.

Townsend, P. and Davidson, N. (1982), *Inequalities in Health-The Black Report*, Penguin:Harmondsworth.

Tudge, C. (1983), *The Food Connection*, BBC:London.

Turner, M. and Gray, J. (1982), *The Implementation of Dietary Guidelines:Obstacles and Opportunities*, British Nutrition Foundation:London.

Turner, A. (1981), "Product Liability and the Food Manufacturer", FDIC Bulletin, 19 November, 18-26. *in*, Grant, W. (1983), *The UK Food Processing Industry*, International Institute of Management:Berlin.

Turner, R. *General Practitioner*, 2nd December,1983.

Turner, R. (1983b), "Of Frail Hearts and Sacred Cows." *The Health Services*, No.44 pp10-11.

Veitch, A. (1985), "Nutritionist's threat to quit over "censorship"", *The Guardian*, 5th August.

Veitch, A.(1986), "Survey on "chips and biscuits" diet to be released" *The Guardian*, April 4 1986.

Veitch, A. and Hencke, D. (1987), "Health education deputy drink, tobacco link", *The Guardian* 19th February.

Vogel, D. (1987), "Political Science and the Study of Corporate Power: A Dissent from the New Conventional Wisdom." *British Journal of Political Science*, Vol. 17, p385-408.

Walker, C. and Cannon, G. (1985), *The Food Scandal*, Century:London.

Walker, C. L., Church, M.B., (1978), "Poverty by administration:a review of supplementary benefits, nutrition and scale rates." *Journal of Human Nutrition* Vol. 32, p5-18.

209

Ward, P. D. (1979), "Health Lobbies:Vested Interests and Pressure Politics", *in*, Cater, D. and Lee, P.R. *Politics of Health*, Robert. E. Kreiger Publishing Co:New York.

Ward, H. (1987), "Structural Power-A Contradiction in Terms?" Political Studies XXXV, p593-610.

Welin, L. (1983) "Why the Incidence of IHD in Sweden is Increasing." The Lancet, No.8333, p1087-1089.

Wenlock, R., Disselduff, M., Skinner, R. and Knight, I, (1986), "The Diets of British Schoolchildren." DHSS:London.

Wheelock, V. and Fallows, S., (1985), "The Implications of the COMA Report on Diet and Cardiovascular Disease for British Agriculture." Food Policy Research:University of Bradford.

Wilks, S. and Wright, M. (eds) (1987), *Comparative Government-Industry Relations*, Clarendon Press:Oxford.

Wilson, G.K. (1977), *Special Interests and Policy Making: Agricultural Policies and Politics in Britain and the United States of America, 1956-70*, John Wiley and Sons:London.

Winikoff, B. (1977), "Nutrition and Food Policy: The Approaches of Norway and the United States", American Journal of Public Health, Vol.67, No.6.

Winnifrith, Sir J. (1962), *The Ministry of Agriculture, Fisheries and Food*, HMSO:London.

Wistow, G. (1989), "The Health Service Policy Community:Professionals Pre-Eminent or Under Challenge?, Paper to the Policy Networks Conference, University of Essex, June 30-July 1.

Wistow, G., and Rhodes, R.A.W., (1987), "Policy Networks and the Policy Process", Paper to the PSA Conference, Aberdeen.

World Health Organisation, (1982), *Prevention of Coronary Heart Disease*, Report of a WHO Expert Committee, Technical Report Series No.678, WHO:Geneva.

World in Action, (1984), "Countdown to a Coronary," Granada TV.

Wright, M., (1987), "Policy Community, Policy Network and Comparative Industrial Policies." Paper to the PSA Conference, Aberdeen.

Index